Pediatric Evidence

The Practice-Changing Studies

Lindsay P. Carter, MD

Instructor in Pediatrics
Harvard Medical School
Division of Pediatric Hospitalist Medicine
Director, Pediatric Advanced Clerkship
Associate Director, Pediatric Core Clerkship
MassGeneral Hospital for Children
Boston, Massachusetts

Meredith G. A. Eicken, MD

Instructor in Medicine
Harvard Medical School
Departments of Medicine and Pediatrics
Massachusetts General Hospital
MassGeneral Hospital for Children
Kraft Fellowship in Community Health
  Leadership
MGH Revere Health Care Center
Boston, Massachusetts

Vandana L. Madhavan, MD, MPH

Instructor in Pediatrics
Harvard Medical School
Divisions of Pediatric Infectious Disease
  and Pediatric Hospitalist Medicine
Pediatric Group Practice
MassGeneral Hospital for Children
Boston, Massachusetts

SERIES EDITORS

Emily L. Aaronson, MD
Erik L. Antonsen, MD, PhD
Arjun K. Venkatesh, MD, MBA, MHS

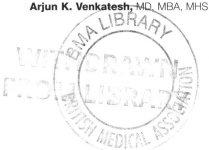

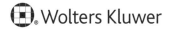. Wolters Kluwer

Philadelphia • Baltimore • New York • Lo
Buenos Aires • Hong Kong • Sydney • To

Acquisitions Editor: Jamie M. Elfrank
Product Development Editor: Ashley Fischer
Editorial Assistant: Brian Convery
Marketing Manager: Stephanie Kindlick
Production Project Manager: David Saltzberg
Design Coordinator: Holly Reid McLaughlin
Manufacturing Coordinator: Beth Welsh
Prepress Vendor: Aptara, Inc.

9 8 7 6 5 4 3 2

Printed in China

Library of Congress Cataloging-in-Publication Data

Names: Carter, Lindsay P., editor. | Eicken, Meredith G. A., editor. |
 Madhavan, Vandana L., editor.
Title: Pediatric evidence : the practice-changing studies / [edited by]
 Lindsay P. Carter, Meredith G. A. Eicken, Vandana L. Madhavan.
Description: Philadelphia : Wolters Kluwer, [2016]
Identifiers: LCCN 2015042927 | ISBN 9781496333315 (paperback)
Subjects: | MESH: Pediatrics–methods. | Clinical Trials as Topic. |
 Evidence-Based Medicine.
Classification: LCC RJ61 | NLM WS 200 | DDC 618.92–dc23
LC record available at http://lccn.loc.gov/2015042927

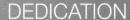

**To my parents Frank and Suzanne Pindyck,
my husband Bill, and my boys Luke and Finn,
who have provided staunch support, unconditional
love, and endless laughter.**

—Lindsay P. Carter, MD

**To my parents Robert and Teresa Albin, who inspired
and encouraged me on this path, and my husband
John, my rock.**

—Meredith G. A. Eicken, MD

**To all of my teachers, in medicine and in life,
especially my parents, C. K. and Deepa Madhavan,
my husband Parag Amin, and our boys Raj and Jay.**

—Vandana L. Madhavan, MD, MPH

**Thank you to our patients who inspire us to continue
expanding our knowledge and to the families who
grant us the privilege of caring for their children.**

CONTRIBUTORS

Mary Perry Alexander, MD, MPH
Resident
Department of Pediatrics
MassGeneral Hospital for Children
Boston, Massachusetts

Lauren Allister, MD
Instructor in Pediatrics
Harvard Medical School
Department of Emergency Medicine
Massachusetts General Hospital
Boston, Massachusetts

Sara V. Bates, MD
Instructor in Pediatrics
Harvard Medical School
Division of Newborn Medicine
MassGeneral Hospital for Children
Boston, Massachusetts

Carolyn Murphy Boscia, MD
Resident
Departments of Medicine and Pediatrics
Massachusetts General Hospital
MassGeneral Hospital for Children
Boston, Massachusetts

Lindsay P. Carter, MD
Instructor in Pediatrics
Harvard Medical School
Division of Pediatric Hospitalist Medicine
Director, Pediatric Advanced Clerkship
Associate Director, Pediatric Core
   Clerkship
MassGeneral Hospital for Children
Boston, Massachusetts

Rebecca Cook, MD, MSc
Chief Resident
Department of Pediatrics
MassGeneral Hospital for Children
Boston, Massachusetts

Brian M. Cummings, MD
Assistant Professor of Pediatrics
Harvard Medical School
Division of Pediatric Critical Care
MassGeneral Hospital for Children
Boston, Massachusetts

Meredith G. A. Eicken, MD
Instructor in Medicine
Harvard Medical School
Departments of Medicine and Pediatrics
Massachusetts General Hospital
MassGeneral Hospital for Children
Kraft Fellowship in Community Health
   Leadership
MGH Revere Health Care Center
Boston, Massachusetts

Chadi M. El Saleeby, MD
Assistant Professor of Pediatrics
Harvard Medical School
Divisions of Pediatric Hospitalist Medicine
   and Pediatric Infectious Disease
MassGeneral Hospital for Children
Boston, Massachusetts

Michael Epstein, MD
Resident
Department of Pediatrics
MassGeneral Hospital for Children
Boston, Massachusetts

Laura Diane Flannery, MD
Resident
Departments of Medicine and Pediatrics
Massachusetts General Hospital
MassGeneral Hospital for Children
Boston, Massachusetts

Matthew G. Gartland, MD
Resident
Departments of Medicine and Pediatrics
Massachusetts General Hospital
MassGeneral Hospital for Children
Boston, Massachusetts

Emily M. Herzberg, MD
Resident
Department of Pediatrics
MassGeneral Hospital for Children
Boston, Massachusetts

Thomas F. Heyne, MD, MSt
Resident
Departments of Medicine and Pediatrics
Massachusetts General Hospital
MassGeneral Hospital for Children
Boston, Massachusetts

Manuella Lahoud-Rahme, MD
Instructor in Pediatrics
Harvard Medical School
Divisions of Pediatric Cardiology and
    Pediatric Critical Care Medicine
MassGeneral Hospital for Children
Boston, Massachusetts

Tanya M. Laidlaw, MD
Assistant Professor of Medicine
Harvard Medical School
Division of Rheumatology, Immunology,
    and Allergy
Brigham and Women's Hospital
Boston, Massachusetts

Vandana L. Madhavan, MD, MPH
Instructor in Pediatrics
Harvard Medical School
Divisions of Pediatric Infectious Disease
    and Pediatric Hospitalist Medicine
Pediatric Group Practice
MassGeneral Hospital for Children
Boston, Massachusetts

Juliana Mariani, MD
Resident
Department of Pediatrics
MassGeneral Hospital for Children
Boston, Massachusetts

Eli M. Miloslavsky, MD
Instructor in Medicine
Harvard Medical School
Division of Rheumatology
Massachusetts General Hospital
Boston, Massachusetts

Molly Miloslavsky, MD
Chief Resident
Department of Pediatrics
MassGeneral Hospital for Children
Boston, Massachusetts

Christopher J. Moran, MD
Instructor in Pediatrics
Harvard Medical School
Division of Pediatric Gastroenterology
    and Nutrition
MassGeneral Hospital for Children
Boston, Massachusetts

Benjamin A. Nelson, MD
Instructor in Pediatrics
Harvard Medical School
Division of Pediatric Pulmonology
MassGeneral Hospital for Children
Boston, Massachusetts

Jenna O'Connell, MD
Resident
Department of Pediatrics
MassGeneral Hospital for Children
Boston, Massachusetts

Marianna S. Parker, MBBS
Fellow
Harvard Neonatal-Perinatal Medicine
    Program
Boston, Massachusetts

Elizabeth Pinsky, MD
Instructor in Pediatrics
Harvard Medical School
Department of Child Psychiatry
Massachusetts General Hospital
Boston, Massachusetts

Max Rubinstein, MD
Fellow in Pediatric Emergency Medicine
The Warren Alpert Medical School of
    Brown University
Department of Pediatric Emergency
    Medicine
Hasbro Children's Hospital
Providence, Rhode Island

Rachel S. Sagor, MD
Department of Pediatrics
Boston University School of Medicine
Boston Medical Center
Boston, Massachusetts

Kevin J. Staley, MD
Joseph P. and Rose F. Kennedy Professor of
    Child Neurology and Mental Retardation
Harvard Medical School
Unit Chief, Pediatric Neurology
Department of Neurology
Massachusetts General Hospital
MassGeneral Hospital for Children
Boston, Massachusetts

Takara Stanley, MD
Assistant Professor of Pediatrics
Harvard Medical School
Division of Pediatric Endocrinology
MassGeneral Hospital for Children
Boston, Massachusetts

Eliza Gardiner Stensland, MD
Resident
Department of Pediatrics
MassGeneral Hospital for Children
Boston, Massachusetts

Patricia Ann Stoeck, MD
Assistant in Medicine
Children's Hospital Inpatient Service
Boston Children's Hospital
Boston, Massachusetts

David A. Sweetser, MD, PhD
Assistant Professor of Pediatrics
Harvard Medical School
Chief of Medical Genetics
Massachusetts General Hospital
Division of Pediatric Hematology/Oncology
MassGeneral Hospital for Children
Boston, Massachusetts

Avram Z. Traum, MD
Instructor in Pediatrics
Harvard Medical School
Division of Nephrology
Boston Children's Hospital
Boston, Massachusetts

Katherine Sheffer Larabee Tuttle, MD
Resident
Department of Pediatrics
MassGeneral Hospital for Children
Boston, Massachusetts

Melissa A. Walker, MD, PhD
Child Neurology Resident
Department of Neurology
Massachusetts General Hospital
Boston, Massachusetts

Howard J. Weinstein, MD
R. Alan Ezekowitz Professor of Pediatrics
Harvard Medical School
Chief, Pediatric Hematology-Oncology
MassGeneral Hospital for Children
Boston, Massachusetts

Elisabeth B. Winterkorn, MD
Instructor in Pediatrics
Harvard Medical School
Private Practice Pediatrics
North Andover, Massachusetts

Lila Worden, MD
Child Neurology Resident
Department of Neurology
Massachusetts General Hospital
Boston, Massachusetts

Kathryn E. Wynne, MD
Assistant Professor of Pediatrics
University of Massachusetts Medical School
Pediatric Hospitalist
Department of Pediatrics
UMass Memorial Children's Medical Center
Worcester, Massachusetts

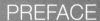

The practice of pediatric medicine can feel very personal; there is an incomprehensible level of trust placed by parents in pediatric providers caring for their children and the enormity of this responsibility is felt by all. We seek to do what is best, but how do we achieve this consistently, especially in the face of ever-changing practice? We believe this endeavor is most successful with the integration of clinical expertise, patient and family preferences, and empiric evidence. However, this is easier in theory than practice, as the body of literature grows at an exponential rate. There are over 195,000 active studies (over 41,000 involving pediatric-aged patients) registered at ClinicalTrials.gov and hundreds of thousands of articles registered at PubMed annually. This sheer volume of data can easily overwhelm trainees or even established providers, but without knowledge of the existing evidence, we cannot effectively practice or counsel patients and families.

As medical students and residents, we were often left wondering about the evidence behind the clinical decision making we witnessed and learned, or whether there was evidence at all. Many of us could quote the "Rochester criteria" for febrile neonates, but few knew the study specifics. Now, as attending physicians, we find ourselves searching the literature regularly to support our care plans or devise new ones. Literature searches can be time consuming and overwhelming, and once a seemingly relevant paper is finally identified, the interpretation and application of data must be individualized to the patient. By discussing some of the most influential original research studies in pediatrics, this book seeks to make the evidence more accessible and provide context for current practice.

In this book, we have compiled and summarized 100 practice-changing articles in the field of pediatrics. There is a mix of historical and contemporary studies, emphasizing the most relevant data for today's practice. Additionally, as select pediatric clinical practices are extrapolated from adult data, there are adult studies included. We acknowledge that, in some areas, there are newer studies or multiple contemporary papers researching the same topics, but each chosen article has something unique to offer. Each has limitations affecting the data and the generalizability of the results, and we have attempted to highlight these, as we believe it is important to recognize when the data fall short so that practitioners are fully informed in choosing a certain treatment course. The question of applicability is vital to practicing evidence-based medicine—do the results apply to the population being cared for?

These articles were chosen systematically and incorporated the expert opinion of MassGeneral Hospital *for* Children faculty. We realize the list is not comprehensive; in truth, each pediatric subspecialty could compile 100 practice-changing articles individually.

We also recognize that within the limited scope of this book, we were not able to adequately address several major contributors to the global burden of pediatric disease and that our focus is on more resourced settings. But we offer these as a starting point. Furthermore, we hope that the commentary highlights the context and importance of each study. There are also references to additional research and guidelines that build upon or support the study reviewed.

We realize that not everyone will agree with our selection and we put forth that another list of 100 could be generated rather easily. We welcome the debate as it means people are discussing the evidence which is our primary goal.

The evidence will continue to evolve at an ever-growing rate. For now, we hope that whether you are a new medical student on your pediatrics rotation or a seasoned provider, this book provides insight into and understanding of today's clinical practice of pediatrics.

Lindsay P. Carter, MD
Meredith G. A. Eicken, MD
Vandana L. Madhavan, MD, MPH

ACKNOWLEDGMENTS

The editors of this book are indebted to many people who helped in this process. We would like to specifically thank Drs. Angela Jacques and Aura Obando, co-creators of a departmental publication entitled *Pediatric PubList* which served as the foundation for this project. We would also like to thank the MassGeneral Hospital *for* Children faculty who helped us formulate a long list of articles to consider for inclusion. We would like to especially thank Drs. Lauren Allister, Brian Cummings, Ann Kao, Sigmund Kharasch, Bernard Kinane, Mark Pasternack, and Gary Russell for their assistance in distilling down the hundreds of papers to the list that appears here. Of course, many thanks to the residents and faculty who wrote and edited the following chapters, providing their expertise and critical appraisal.

CONTENTS

SECTION 1: ALLERGY/IMMUNOLOGY

Resident Author: Katherine S. L. Tuttle
Faculty Author: Tanya M. Laidlaw

1. Oral Immunotherapy for Egg Allergy Desensitization 2
2. Clinical Identification of Primary Immunodeficiency 4
3. Cow's Milk Allergy 6
4. Peanut Allergy 8
5. Biphasic Reactions in Anaphylaxis 10

SECTION 2: CARDIOLOGY

Resident Author: Laura Flannery
Faculty Author: Manuella Lahoud-Rahme

6. Causes of Chest Pain 14
7. Newborn Screening with Pulse Oximetry 18
8. Identification of Fetuses at Risk for Hypoplastic Left Heart
Syndrome 20
9. Impact of Weight on Outcomes in Repair of Congenital
Heart Defects 22
10. Sudden Death in Young Athletes 24

SECTION 3: CRITICAL CARE

Resident Authors: Carolyn Murphy Boscia, Matthew G. Gartland
Faculty Author: Brian M. Cummings

11. Early Antibiotics in Pediatric Sepsis 28
12. Interruption of Sedation for Early Extubation 30
13. Bundled Care for Reduction of Central Line Infections 32

14. High-Flow Nasal Cannula for Bronchiolitis.. 34
15. Bystander CPR in Pediatric Out-of-Hospital Cardiac Arrest 36
16. Restrictive Protocol for Blood Transfusions 38
17. Low Tidal Volume Ventilation in Acute Respiratory Distress Syndrome ... 40
18. Early Fluid Resuscitation in Septic Shock... 42

SECTION 4: EMERGENCY MEDICINE
Resident Authors: Emily M. Herzberg, Thomas F. Heyne
Faculty Author: Lauren Allister

19. A Prediction Rule for Appendicitis... 46
20. Need for CT Scan in Head Trauma... 48
21. Utility of Lumbar Puncture in First Simple Febrile Seizure.................. 52
22. Oral Ondansetron for Gastroenteritis... 54
23. Oral versus Intravenous Rehydration... 56
24. Oral Dexamethasone for Mild Croup.. 58
25. Likelihood of Occult Pneumonia in Febrile Children........................... 60
26. Ipratropium in Acute Asthma Management... 62
27. Evaluation of the Febrile Infant 64

SECTION 5: ENDOCRINOLOGY
Resident Author: Mary Perry Alexander
Faculty Author: Takara Stanley

28. Maintenance of Glycemic Control in Type 2 Diabetes 70
29. Impact of Body Mass Index on Pubertal Development 72
30. Cerebral Edema in Diabetic Ketoacidosis 74
31. Intensive Insulin Treatment for Type 1 Diabetes................................ 76
32. Prevention of Intellectual Impairment with Neonatal Hypothyroidism
Screening 78

SECTION 6: GASTROENTEROLOGY
Resident Author: Kathryn E. Wynne
Faculty Author: Christopher J. Moran

33. Introduction of Gluten and Celiac Disease Risk.................................. 82
34. Use of PUCAI Score in Ulcerative Colitis.. 84

35. Infliximab Therapy for Crohn's Disease... 86

36. Prevalence of Celiac Disease 88

37. Polyethylene Glycol Treatment for Constipation 90

SECTION 7: GENETICS

Resident Author: Lila Worden

Faculty Author: David A. Sweetser

38. Whole-Exome Sequencing... 94

39. Noninvasive Prenatal Testing for Trisomy 21 96

40. Mass Spectrometry Screening for Inborn Errors of Metabolism 98

41. Angiotensin Receptor Blockade in Marfan Syndrome 100

SECTION 8: HEMATOLOGY/ONCOLOGY

Resident Authors: Juliana Mariani, Patricia A. Stoeck

Faculty Author: Howard J. Weinstein

42. Genetic Predictors of Unfavorable Outcomes in Pediatric
Medulloblastoma 104

43. Prophylactic Treatment with Factor VIII in Hemophilia 108

44. Significance of Minimal Residual Disease in Acute
Lymphoblastic Leukemia 110

45. Increased Incidence of Chronic Disease in Survivors of
Childhood Cancer.. 112

46. Treatment of Acute Idiopathic Thrombocytopenic Purpura................ 114

47. Hydroxyurea Therapy in Sickle Cell Anemia 116

48. Symptom Management at the End of Life in Pediatric Oncology 118

49. Stroke Risk Reduction in Sickle Cell Anemia.................................. 120

SECTION 9: INFECTIOUS DISEASES

Resident Authors: Rebecca Cook, Matthew G. Gartland,
Thomas F. Heyne, Juliana Mariani, Molly Miloslavsky

Faculty Author: Chadi M. El Saleeby

50. Management of Community-Acquired Skin Abscesses..................... 124

51. Sequential Therapy in the Treatment of Osteomyelitis 126

52. Impact of Antibiotic Pretreatment on Cerebrospinal Fluid Profiles....... 128

53. Concomitant Bacterial Infection in Infants with Respiratory
Syncytial Virus 130

54. High-Dose Acyclovir for Neonatal Herpes Simplex Virus Infection 132

55. Clinical Prediction Algorithm for Septic Arthritis 134

56. Oral versus Intravenous Therapy for Urinary Tract Infections 136

57. Palivizumab for Reduction of Respiratory Syncytial Virus Infections ... 138

58. Reduction in Mother-to-Child Transmission of Human
Immunodeficiency Virus 140

SECTION 10: NEONATOLOGY

Resident Authors: Rebecca Cook, Marianna Parker
Faculty Author: Sara V. Bates

59. Predictors for Survival in Extreme Prematurity 144

60. Caffeine for Apnea of Prematurity 146

61. Therapeutic Hypothermia in Hypoxic-Ischemic Encephalopathy 148

62. Reduction of Group B Streptococcal Disease 150

63. Management of the Meconium-Stained Neonate 152

64. Bilirubin Screening in Neonates 154

65. Surfactant in Respiratory Distress Syndrome 158

SECTION 11: NEUROLOGY

Resident Author: Melissa A. Walker
Faculty Author: Kevin J. Staley

66. Seizure Recurrence after Withdrawal of Antiepileptic Drugs 162

67. Developmental Outcomes after Preterm Births 164

68. Serious Intracranial Pathology in Chronic Headache 166

69. Amitriptyline in Migraine Prophylaxis 168

70. Risk of Unprovoked Seizures after Febrile Seizures 170

SECTION 12: PRIMARY CARE

Resident Authors: Jenna M. O'Connell, Rachel S. Sagor, Eliza G. Stensland
Faculty Author: Elisabeth B. Winterkorn

71. Long-Acting Reversible Contraception in Adolescents 174

72. Treatment of Acute Otitis Media 176

73. Childhood Obesity and Cardiovascular Risk 178

74. Sexually Transmitted Infection Prevalence.. 180

75. Cold Medication for Nocturnal Cough in Children 182

76. Effect of Low-Level Lead Exposure on Intellectual Impairment........... 184

77. Measles, Mumps, and Rubella Vaccination and Autism 186

78. Risk of Sudden Infant Death Syndrome with Sleeping Factors........... 188

SECTION 13: PSYCHIATRY/DEVELOPMENT

Resident Authors: Rachel S. Sagor, Lila Worden
Faculty Author: Elizabeth Pinsky

79. Medications versus Cognitive Behavioral Therapy in the
Treatment of Depression.. 192

80. Medication versus Behavioral Treatment in Attention Deficit
Hyperactivity Disorder.. 194

81. Childhood Psychosocial Stress and Adult Disease 198

82. Effect of Early Developmental Intervention in Preterm Infants............. 200

83. Behavioral Intervention for Autism.. 202

SECTION 14: PULMONOLOGY

Resident Authors: Max Rubinstein, Eliza G. Stensland
Faculty Author: Benjamin A. Nelson

84. Adenotonsillectomy for Obstructive Sleep Apnea............................... 206

85. Hypertonic Saline in Cystic Fibrosis 208

86. Budesonide Treatment for Mild Asthma 210

87. Comparison of Oral Corticosteroid Doses in Asthma......................... 212

88. Albuterol, Epinephrine, and Normal Saline for Bronchiolitis 214

89. Impact of Newborn Screening on Nutritional Status in Cystic Fibrosis... 216

90. Route of Delivery of Beta-Agonist Therapy 218

91. Risk of Asthma in Children with Early Wheezing 220

SECTION 15: RENAL

Resident Authors: Michael Epstein
Faculty Author: Avram Z. Traum

92. Antimicrobial Prophylaxis for Children with Vesicoureteral Reflux........ 224

93. Mortality Associated with Acute Kidney Injury 226

94. Impact of Blood Pressure Control on Progression of
Renal Failure 228

95. Outcomes after Acute Kidney Injury 230

96. Response to Prednisone in Nephrotic Syndrome 232

SECTION 16: RHEUMATOLOGY

Resident Author: Molly Miloslavsky
Faculty Author: Eli Miloslavsky

97. Anakinra in Systemic Juvenile Idiopathic Arthritis 236

98. Treatment of Lupus with Mycophenolate Mofetil 238

99. Etanercept in Treatment of Juvenile Idiopathic Arthritis 240

100. Intravenous Immune Globulin for Kawasaki Disease 242

INDEX 245

STANDARD ABBREVIATIONS

mg   milligram

g   gram

kg   kilogram

CT   computed tomography

GI   gastrointestinal

PO   per os, (i.e., oral)

IV   intravenous

CI   confidence interval

PPV   positive predictive value

NPV   negative predictive value

OR   odds ratio

RR   relative risk

LR   likelihood ratio

ALLERGY/ IMMUNOLOGY

1. Oral Immunotherapy for Egg Allergy Desensitization
2. Clinical Identification of Primary Immunodeficiency
3. Cow's Milk Allergy
4. Peanut Allergy
5. Biphasic Reactions in Anaphylaxis

CHAPTER 1

ORAL IMMUNOTHERAPY FOR EGG ALLERGY DESENSITIZATION

Katherine S. L. Tuttle ■ Tanya M. Laidlaw

Oral Immunotherapy for Treatment of Egg Allergy in Children

Burks AW, Jones SM, Wood RA, et al; Consortium of Food Allergy Research (CoFAR). *N Engl J Med.* 2012;367(3):233–243

BACKGROUND

Avoidance is the only currently recommended therapy for food allergy, although it is fraught with challenges. Recently, oral immunotherapy (OIT) showed efficacy in desensitizing milk and peanut allergic children in small studies, but the safety and efficacy of OIT for egg allergy was previously unknown.

OBJECTIVES

To examine the efficacy and safety of egg OIT to induce "sustained unresponsiveness" (ability to consume 10 g egg-white powder and a cooked egg without significant symptoms after egg avoidance for 4 to 6 weeks) and "desensitization" (ability to pass an oral food challenge [OFC] while receiving daily OIT) in children with egg allergy.

METHODS

Double-blind, randomized, placebo-controlled trial in 5 US centers from 2007 to 2010.

Patients

55 children ages 5 to 11 years with egg allergy and egg-specific Immunoglobulin (Ig) E levels greater than 5 kU/L for children >6 years or 12 kU/L for 5-year-olds. Select exclusion criteria: corn allergy, severe asthma, or history of severe anaphylaxis to egg.

Intervention

Children received placebo (cornstarch) or egg OIT increased up to 2 g per day. After 10 months, maintenance OFC was performed. The study was then unblinded and the placebo treatment was stopped but OIT was continued. Repeat OFC was performed at 22 months; those who passed that OFC stopped OIT and avoided eggs for 4 to 6 weeks. Subsequent OFC with 10 g egg-white powder and a cooked egg was done at 24 months to test for sustained unresponsiveness; those who passed then advanced to egg ad libitum diet with reassessments at 30 and 36 months. Skin prick testing and egg-white-specific IgE and IgG4 levels were measured periodically.

Outcomes

Primary outcome was induction of sustained unresponsiveness after 22 months of egg OIT. Secondary outcomes included desensitization and safety.

KEY RESULTS

- 11/40 (28%) children receiving OIT developed sustained unresponsiveness as compared to 0/15 (0%) receiving placebo ($p = 0.03$).
- 22/40 (55%) children receiving egg OIT and 0/15 (0%) on placebo were desensitized at 10 months ($p < 0.001$). This increased to 30/40 (75%) children on OIT at 22 months ($p < 0.001$), all of whom continued to eat egg 1 year out.
- Most common adverse event was oropharyngeal symptoms, seen in 25% of egg OIT doses and 3.9% of placebo doses ($p < 0.001$), but this improved after 10 months.

STUDY CONCLUSIONS

Egg OIT was safe and induced sustained unresponsiveness even after a period of egg avoidance off OIT in 28% of children. Desensitization was achieved in up to 75% of children on OIT.

COMMENTARY

This study detailed the capacity to achieve desensitization and sustained unresponsiveness to egg through prolonged OIT. OIT is an exciting and promising treatment for egg allergy for a subset of children. On a population level, even if not able to achieve sustained unresponsiveness, desensitization afforded by OIT offers protection from severe reactions with accidental ingestion. Oropharyngeal symptoms were observed frequently in patients dosed with OIT in this study, which may hinder adherence in clinical practice. Larger studies are needed to evaluate OIT use in other food allergies and observe long-term outcomes after cessation of OIT; however, this offers a potential alternative to dietary avoidance as treatment for food allergy in children.

Question

Is OIT a safe and effective treatment for egg allergy?

Answer

Yes, for a subset of children, egg OIT is effective at inducing clinical tolerance. Oropharyngeal symptoms are the most common adverse events during OIT.

CLINICAL IDENTIFICATION OF PRIMARY IMMUNODEFICIENCY

CHAPTER 2

Katherine S. L. Tuttle ■ Tanya M. Laidlaw

Clinical Features That Identify Children With Primary Immunodeficiency Diseases
Subbarayan A, Colarusso G, Hughes SM, et al. *Pediatrics.* 2011;127(5):810–816

BACKGROUND

Primary immunodeficiency diseases (PID) comprise over 200 individual conditions. Although quite rare in the US population, a delay in diagnosis may be associated with increased morbidity due to life-threatening infections. Many US states test for some PIDs on newborn screens; however, not all immunodeficiencies will be detected. Therefore, patient advocacy groups are championing an expert opinion–derived diagnostic schema entitled "10 Warning Signs of PID" in order to increase awareness of these conditions. These signs include: (1) ≥4 ear infections within 1 year, (2) ≥2 serious sinus infections within 1 year, (3) ≥2 months of oral antibiotic treatment with little effect, (4) ≥2 episodes of pneumonia within 1 year, (5) failure to thrive, (6) recurrent deep skin or organ abscesses, (7) persistent thrush or fungal skin infection, (8) need for IV antibiotics, (9) ≥2 deep-seated infections, including sepsis, and (10) family history of PID. This study sought to rigorously evaluate the diagnostic efficacy of this schema.

OBJECTIVES

To determine which of the 10 warning signs best identify children with PID and assess what awareness campaigns should target.

METHODS

Retrospective cohort study at 2 regional pediatric immunology centers in England from 2000 to 2010.

Patients

430 children with a defined PID (categorized as T-cell, B-cell, complement, or neutrophil) and 133 control children with severe, unusual, or recurrent infections with no identifiable specific PID. Select exclusion criteria: none.

Intervention

Comparison of the relative frequency and predictive value of the 10 warning signs of PID.

Outcomes

Primary outcomes were frequency of 10 warning signs and their predictive value. Secondary factors were demographic data, age, and diagnosis.

KEY RESULTS

- Positive family history, failure to thrive, and need for IV antibiotics to clear infections identified 96% of the study population with neutrophil or complement PID and 89% with T-cell PID.
- Family history of physician-diagnosed PID was the strongest identifier of PID overall (RR 18, 95% CI 8–45), and the only identifier of complement PID (RR 142, 95% CI 20–999).
- Family history (RR 8, 95% CI 3–22) and ≥2 months of oral antibiotic treatment with little effect (RR 11, 95% CI 2–48) were the only identifiers of B-cell PID.
- 95% (536) of patients with PID or recurrent infections were referred by hospital-based pediatricians.

STUDY CONCLUSIONS

Family history of PID, need for IV antibiotics to treat infections, and failure to thrive were the most predictive factors in identifying children with PID. Education on clinical identifiers of PID should target hospital-based pediatricians and families of children with PID.

COMMENTARY

This study tested an algorithm for identifying PID based on the expert opinion-derived warning signs, and highlighted the 3 most predictive: family history, need for IV antibiotics to clear infections, and failure to thrive. Of note, it was conducted in a non-US population and no general pediatric control group was analyzed; further studies are therefore needed to validate these results in the general population of US children. Nonetheless, this study emphasizes the importance of eliciting a detailed family and growth history in a patient with recurrent infections, as embarking on a complex investigation without these warning signs may be unwarranted. Patients with complement or B-cell PID are difficult to differentiate based on clinical history necessitating a lower threshold for laboratory investigation.

Question

Are there evidence-based warning signs for PID?

Answer

Family history, failure to thrive, and need for IV antibiotics to clear infections identifies nearly 90% of the patients with primary T-cell, complement, and neutrophil immunodeficiencies.

CHAPTER 3

COW'S MILK ALLERGY

Katherine S. L. Tuttle ■ Tanya M. Laidlaw

The Natural History of IgE-Mediated Cow's Milk Allergy

Skripak JM, Matsui EC, Mudd K, et al. *J Allergy Clin Immunol.* 2007;120(5): 1172–1177

BACKGROUND

Cow's milk allergy (CMA) affects approximately 2% of US children.[1] The largest study to date found that 75% of children with Immunoglobulin (Ig) E–mediated CMA were able to tolerate milk by 3 years of age.[2] However, there are little data to help predict which patients will outgrow this allergy.

OBJECTIVES

To define the clinical course and resolution rate of CMA in children and identify the clinical and laboratory features that predict development of tolerance to cow's milk.

METHODS

Retrospective chart review at 2 US pediatric allergy clinics from 1993 to 2007.

Patients

807 patients ages 13 months to 17 years with IgE-mediated CMA. Select exclusion criteria: non–IgE-mediated disease and only 1 recorded visit.

Intervention

Review of clinical history, outcomes, and test results for children with CMA and comparison of tolerance acquisition rates utilizing various cutoffs from food challenges and cow's milk IgE levels.

Outcomes

Primary outcome was acquisition of oral tolerance to cow's milk (defined after analysis as passing an oral food challenge to milk or as having experienced no reactions to milk in the past 12 months and a cow's milk IgE level <3 kU/L). Secondary outcomes assessed for predictive factors including asthma, allergic rhinitis, eczema, and type of feeding (breast vs. formula).

KEY RESULTS

- CMA resolution rates using the above criteria were 19% by age 4 (95% CI 16–22), 42% by age 8 (95% CI 39–47), 64% by age 12 (95% CI 59–70), and 79% by age 16 (95% CI 72–86).
- Children with persistent CMA had higher median cow's milk IgE levels in the first 2 years of life than those with resolved allergy (19 vs. 1.8 kU/L, $p < 0.001$).
- At ages 4, 8, and 12, asthma and allergic rhinitis were negative predictors for achieving tolerance ($p < 0.0001$); atopic dermatitis, other food allergies, sex, and breast-feeding history were not predictive.

STUDY CONCLUSIONS

Children achieved tolerance to cow's milk later than previously reported, extending into adolescence. Degree of cow's milk IgE elevation was predictive of outcome.

COMMENTARY

This study was the first to describe low rates of CMA resolution, contradicting previous findings.[2] It also highlighted negative predictors for allergy resolution including high-peak cow's milk IgE, increasing cow's milk IgE over the first 1 to 4 years of life, and the presence of allergic rhinitis or asthma. These findings are a crucial component of prognostic discussions with patients and their families. It is unclear if the older average age at which tolerance was achieved was due to the highly atopic nature of the study's referral population (as the authors speculate), or if CMA is evolving into a more complex and chronic disease than previously thought.

Question

Can we predict which children with cow's milk allergy will outgrow their allergy and in what time frame?

Answer

Using a definition of passing an oral challenge or having cow's milk–specific IgE <3 kU/L and no history of clinical reactivity in the previous 12 months, only 19% of patients were tolerant by age 4 years, although 79% resolved by age 16. Comorbid asthma and allergic rhinitis, and a high-peak cow's milk IgE were negative predictors of tolerance.

References

1. Sicherer SH, Sampson HA. Food allergy: Epidemiology, pathogenesis, diagnosis and treatment. *J Allergy Clin Immunol.* 2014;133(2):291–307.
2. Host A, Halken S. A prospective study of cow milk allergy in Danish infants during the first 3 years of life. Clinical course in relation to clinical and immunological type of hypersensitivity reaction. *Allergy.* 1990; 45(8):587–596.

CHAPTER 4   PEANUT ALLERGY

Katherine S. L. Tuttle ■ Tanya M. Laidlaw

The Natural Progression of Peanut Allergy: Resolution and Possibility of Recurrence

Fleischer DM, Conover-Walker MK, Christie L, et al. *J Allergy Clin Immunol.* 2003; 112(1):183–189

BACKGROUND

Peanut allergy was once thought to be a lifelong condition, but current literature estimates that 20% of children actually outgrow their allergy.[1] However, there are several reported cases of children who passed an oral peanut challenge (OPC) and later exhibited allergic symptoms to peanut, suggesting ongoing assessment is crucial. This study sought to describe the natural history of peanut allergy to provide accurate prognostic information.

OBJECTIVES

To describe the natural progression of peanut allergy and characterize dietary patterns and allergy recurrence in patients who passed an OPC.

METHODS

Retrospective chart review in 2 US centers from 2000 to 2002.

Patients

Chart review included 84 patients ages 4 to 15 years with peanut allergy and peanut-specific Immunoglobulin (Ig) E levels of <5 kU/L. Survey included 64 patients ages 4 to 20 years who passed an OPC. Select exclusion criteria: history of multiple peanut challenges.

Intervention

Review of 78 open and 6 double-blind placebo-controlled OPCs as well as survey of patients who passed open OPCs. Data were collected on clinical and reaction history, dietary habits, and IgE levels.

Outcomes

Primary outcome was OPC pass rate. Secondary outcomes were percentage of patients eating peanut products, percentage of families reading labels for peanut products, and recurrence of clinical symptoms of peanut allergy after passing an OPC.

KEY RESULTS
- 44 (55%) patients passed OPCs, with higher pass rates (22/30 patients, 73%) in patients with undetectable peanut-specific IgE levels.
- Children with peanut-specific IgE <2 kU/L were more likely to pass an OPC as compared to those with IgE between 2 and 5 kU/L ($p < 0.003$).
- Severity of initial reactions, peanut-specific IgE levels at the time of diagnosis of allergy, history of atopic disorders, and additional food allergies were not predictive of challenge outcome.
- At a median of 1.6 years after passing an OPC, only 18 (28%) patients ate peanut regularly.
- 2 patients had possible reactions to peanut after passing OPCs, suggesting potential allergy recurrence.

STUDY CONCLUSIONS
There was utility in challenging peanut-allergic patients if their peanut-specific IgE levels were <2 kU/L, as most of those patients passed an OPC. However, even after passing a challenge, only 28% of patients regularly ate peanuts.

COMMENTARY
This study supports routine peanut IgE testing to guide timing of OPC. Surprisingly, only 28% of patients ate peanuts regularly after passing OPCs, which has implications for persistence of oral peanut tolerance and allergy recurrence. We recommend consistent peanut ingestion if patients have passed an OPC and continue with low IgE levels to maintain clinical tolerance. Of note, a recent landmark study concluded that early peanut introduction decreased the frequency of peanut allergy in atopic children; future clinical and research foci may therefore shift toward early, consistent introduction of peanut to induce clinical tolerance.[2]

Question
Can a child outgrow a peanut allergy?

Answer
Possibly. Patients with peanut-specific IgE levels of <2 kU/L have a 63% chance of passing a peanut oral challenge, but there is risk of a reaction during challenge even for patients with undetectable peanut IgE, as well as possible future recurrence of peanut allergy.

References
1. Skolnick HS, Conover-Walker MK, Koerner CB, et al. The natural history of peanut allergy. *J Allergy Clin Immunol.* 2001;107(2):367–374.
2. Du Toit G, Roberts G, Sayre PH, et al. Randomized trial of peanut consumption in infants at risk for peanut allergy. *N Engl J Med.* 2015;372(9):803–813.

CHAPTER 5
BIPHASIC REACTIONS IN ANAPHYLAXIS

Katherine S. L. Tuttle ■ Tanya M. Laidlaw

Biphasic Anaphylactic Reactions in Pediatrics

Lee JM, Greenes DS. *Pediatrics.* 2000;106(4):762–766

BACKGROUND
Biphasic reactions can occur 2 to 72 hours after resolution of the initial anaphylactic episode. Therefore, many experts advocate for 8 to 24 hours' observation after an anaphylactic reaction, a recommendation with significant social and economic impact on patients, families, and our healthcare system. Previous investigations in adults had reported that between 5% and 20% of anaphylactic episodes were complicated by a biphasic reaction, but this topic had not been studied in pediatrics.

OBJECTIVES
To assess the incidence of and risk factors for biphasic reactions in children with anaphylaxis, and to determine the utility of inpatient observation after the initial allergic symptoms resolve.

METHODS
Retrospective, unblinded chart review of all children admitted to a large US urban children's hospital from 1985 to 1999.

Patients
106 patients ages 6 months to 21 years with billing discharge codes related to anaphylaxis (acute allergic reaction with involvement of ≥2 organ systems) with 108 anaphylactic episodes. Select exclusion criteria: development of anaphylaxis during unrelated hospitalization, chronic idiopathic anaphylaxis.

Intervention
Estimation of risk factors for biphasic reactions, based on medical record review of history, symptoms, and treatment. Resolution of anaphylaxis was defined as cessation of all symptoms and no therapy needed for 1 hour. Biphasic reactions were categorized as subsequent recurrence of symptoms requiring therapy.

Outcomes
Primary outcome was occurrence of biphasic reaction. Secondary outcomes were anaphylactic trigger, length of hospitalization, time from allergen exposure to anaphylaxis, time to epinephrine administration, time to biphasic reaction, and symptoms of biphasic reaction.

KEY RESULTS

- 83 (77%) cases involved serious anaphylactic symptoms and 2 cases were fatal.
- 96 (89%) cases were treated with epinephrine. The time to initial epinephrine dose was 142 minutes longer for patients with biphasic reactions ($p < 0.03$).
- Biphasic reactions occurred in 6/105 patients (6%); only 2 had serious reactions in the first 24 hours. All had received epinephrine initially, and 5/6 received steroids.
- Median length of inpatient observation was 19 hours (mean 24 ± 21). Time to biphasic reaction from initial symptoms ranged from 5.6 to 47.6 hours.

STUDY CONCLUSIONS

6% of pediatric anaphylactic episodes were complicated by a biphasic reaction. Delayed administration of epinephrine was the only risk factor associated with increased incidence of these biphasic reactions. Only 2% of patients benefited from a 24-hour observation period.

COMMENTARY

This extensive retrospective study demonstrated that the incidence of biphasic reactions is significantly lower than previously thought, and that there is a wide range of time from initial symptoms to onset of biphasic reactions. The only significant risk factor was delayed epinephrine administration, which was also a risk factor in a study of fatal and near-fatal cases of anaphylaxis.[1] This highlights the need to focus on early identification and treatment of anaphylaxis. Given that a 24-hour inpatient observation has significant social and financial impact and would not capture all biphasic reactions, these data support discharge from the ED if epinephrine is promptly given and safe disposition planning is completed.

Question

Do all pediatric patients with anaphylaxis require 24-hour admission to monitor for a biphasic reaction?

Answer

No. Biphasic reactions in children are uncommon, particularly if epinephrine is administered rapidly, and do not always occur within a 24-hour period; therefore there are insufficient data to support this practice.

Reference

1. Sampson HA, Mendelson L, Rosen JP. Fatal and near-fatal anaphylactic reactions to food in children and adolescents. *N Engl J Med.* 1992;327(6):380–384.

CARDIOLOGY

6. Causes of Chest Pain
7. Newborn Screening with Pulse Oximetry
8. Identification of Fetuses at Risk for Hypoplastic Left Heart Syndrome
9. Impact of Weight on Outcomes in Repair of Congenital Heart Defects
10. Sudden Death in Young Athletes

CHAPTER 6 CAUSES OF CHEST PAIN

Laura Flannery ■ Manuella Lahoud-Rahme

Effectiveness of Screening for Life-Threatening Chest Pain in Children
Saleeb SF, Li WY, Warren SZ, et al. *Pediatrics.* 2011;128(5):e1062–e1068

BACKGROUND
Chest pain (CP) accounts for 5% of pediatric cardiology consultations, and nearly 20% of pediatric emergency department cardiology consults for previously unevaluated patients.[1] This symptom triggers a great deal of anxiety and fear, both because CP often reveals a significant problem in adults and because of the rare instances of sudden cardiac death in young people. This leads to excessive referrals and costly evaluations for CP in the pediatric population.

OBJECTIVES
To determine the incidence of cardiac pathology and death from a cardiac condition in patients with CP.

METHODS
Retrospective chart review in a single US center from 2000 to 2009.

Patients
3,700 patients ages 7 to 22 years seen in cardiology clinic for CP. Select exclusion criteria: known significant cardiovascular disease, previous cardiac evaluations for systemic illness or family history of cardiac disease, normal cardiac evaluation for CP at another institution.

Intervention
Records with billing codes for CP assessment and national databases were reviewed for demographic data, clinical features, ancillary cardiac testing, and death records. Median follow-up time after the clinic visit was 4 years.

Outcomes
Primary outcome was cardiac-related death. Secondary outcomes were clinical symptoms, number of cardiac tests, and diagnoses of CP etiology.

KEY RESULTS
- There were 3 deaths, none were cardiac.
- 1% (37) of patients were determined to have a cardiac cause of CP. Other etiologies included musculoskeletal (36%), pulmonary (7%), GI (3%), anxiety (1%), and unknown (52%).
- Of the 37 patients with a cardiac cause of CP, 29 (78%) had a concerning history (e.g., positional or exertional CP, palpitations, family history of congenital heart disease), 12 (32%) had an abnormal electrocardiogram (EKG), and 5 (14%) had an abnormal physical examination finding (e.g., pericardial friction rub or ectopy).
- 1,410 (38%) patients underwent echocardiography, of which only 11 (0.8%) had positive findings potentially explaining CP. Most common diagnoses were anomalous right coronary artery, pericardial effusion, myocarditis, and hypertrophic or dilated cardiomyopathy.
- Exercise stress tests were performed for 769 (21%) patients, of which only 1 (0.1%) had ischemic changes, considered a false positive.
- Rhythm monitors were applied to 1,096 patients (30%) and were positive in 13 patients (0.4%). Supraventricular tachycardia was the most common diagnosis.

STUDY CONCLUSIONS
Only 1% of patients with CP had a cardiac etiology, and no patient who presented to clinic with a complaint of CP died of a cardiac condition.

COMMENTARY
This study demonstrated that CP in children is not often an indication of serious cardiac disease. Importantly, it showed that "red flags" in the history, physical examination, or EKG can help practitioners identify the rare patient with CP who warrants further evaluation. Of note, a large volume of low-yield ancillary testing (echocardiogram, stress tests, and rhythm monitoring) was performed, with an average of 0.8 test per patient presenting with CP with only 1% having positive findings. A subsequent study developed an algorithm to guide clinical decision making surrounding additional testing, with the goal of avoiding low-value or unnecessary testing and referrals (Fig. 6.1).

Question
Likely is CP to be a symptom indicative of serious disease in children?

Answer
It is unlikely; in 99% of the cases, CP in pediatric patients is noncardiac.

Reference

1. Geggel RL. Conditions leading to pediatric cardiology consultation in a tertiary academic hospital. *Pediatrics.* 2004;114(4):e409–e417.

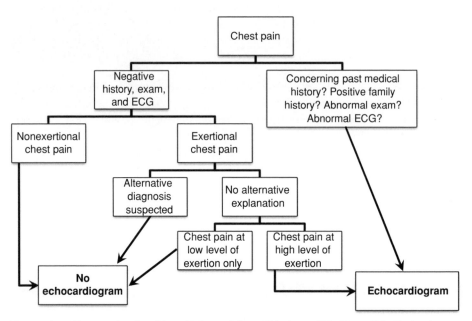

Figure 6.1 Chest pain algorithm. (Adapted from Friedman KG, Kane DA, Rathod RH, et al. Management of pediatric chest pain using a standardized assessment and management plan. *Pediatrics.* 2011;128(2):239–245, Figure 1.)

CHAPTER 7

NEWBORN SCREENING WITH PULSE OXIMETRY

Laura Flannery ■ Manuella Lahoud-Rahme

Pulse Oximetry Screening for Congenital Heart Defects in Newborn Infants (Pulseox): A Test Accuracy Study

Ewer AK, Middleton LJ, Furmston AT, et al. *Lancet.* 2011;378(9793):785–794

BACKGROUND

Congenital heart disease (CHD) is the leading cause of birth defect–associated neonatal death; approximately 6:1,000 newborns have moderate-to-severe CHD.[1] Previously, screening relied on prenatal ultrasounds and newborn examinations which had fairly low detection rates; up to 23% of newborns with severe CHD were discharged undiagnosed, of whom 2% died.[2] This study sought to investigate the benefit of addition of pulse oximetry screening.

OBJECTIVES

To assess the accuracy of pulse oximetry for screening of major CHD and determine additive value beyond prenatal ultrasonography screening.

METHODS

Prospective study in 6 maternity units in the United Kingdom from 2008 to 2009.

Patients

20,055 asymptomatic newborns >34 weeks' gestation, including those with suspected CHD on prenatal ultrasound. Select exclusion criterion: symptoms of cardiac disease.

Intervention

Pulse oximetry screening was performed at <24 hours of age or before discharge. Normal saturation was defined as >95% in right upper and either lower extremity, and discrepancy <2% between the 2 limbs. If oximetry screening was abnormal but clinical examination was normal, oximetry was repeated. If both were abnormal, or there was persistently abnormal oximetry with normal examination, echocardiography was performed as the reference standard. Registries and databases were reviewed to determine later diagnosis of CHD.

Outcomes

Primary outcome was sensitivity and specificity of pulse oximetry for detection of critical CHD (requiring invasive intervention or causing death within 28 days of life) or major CHD (requiring invasive intervention or causing death within 12 months of life).

KEY RESULTS
- 53 infants had major CHD, of which 24 were critical. 26 of these infants had abnormal pulse oximetry.
- Overall, pulse oximetry alone had sensitivities of 75% (95% CI 53–90) and 49% (95% CI 35–63) for critical and major CHD, respectively, compared to prenatal ultrasonography which had 50% (95% CI 29–71) and 36% (95% CI 23–50) sensitivities.
- In the cohort of newborns with no suspicion for CHD on prenatal ultrasound, pulse oximetry had sensitivities of 58% (95% CI 28–85) and 29% (95% CI 15–46%) for critical and major CHD.
- False positives in the first 24 hours of life occurred in 0.8% (169) of newborns, but several had other illnesses requiring intervention (e.g., pneumonia).
- The combined sensitivity of prenatal ultrasound, newborn physical examination, and pulse oximetry was 92% for critical CHD.

STUDY CONCLUSIONS
Pulse oximetry screening was fairly sensitive for detecting major or critical CHD. When added to routine prenatal ultrasonography and postnatal examination, it identified >90% of critical CHD.

COMMENTARY

This study confirmed utility of pulse oximetry as adjunct screening and established optimal timing for screening as >24 hours of life to reduce the false-positive rate. Pulse oximetry is noninvasive, inexpensive, and easily implemented, and was therefore added in 2011 to the US Recommended Uniform Screening Panel for newborns. A subsequent cost-effectiveness analysis estimated that routine oximetry screening would cost an additional $6.28 per newborn and save 20 infant lives annually at a cost of $40,385 per life-year gained.[2]

Question
How helpful is pulse oximetry screening in detecting CHD in newborns?

Answer
Oximetry screening is a simple, noninvasive test; when combined with prenatal ultrasound and postnatal clinical examination, it has a 92% sensitivity for critical CHD.

References
1. Hoffman JI, Kaplan S. The incidence of congenital heart disease. *J Am Coll Cardiol.* 2002;39(12):1890–1900.
2. Peterson C, Grosse SD, Oster ME, et al. Cost-effectiveness of routine screening for critical congenital heart disease in US newborns. *Pediatrics.* 2013;132(3):e595–e603.

CHAPTER 8

IDENTIFICATION OF FETUSES AT RISK FOR HYPOPLASTIC LEFT HEART SYNDROME

Laura Flannery ■ Manuella Lahoud-Rahme

Fetal Aortic Valve Stenosis and the Evolution of Hypoplastic Left Heart Syndrome: Patient Selection for Fetal Intervention

Mäkikallio K, McElhinney DB, Levine JC, et al. *Circulation.* 2006;113(11):1401–1405

BACKGROUND

Management options for hypoplastic left heart syndrome (HLHS) traditionally included staged surgical palliation to a single-ventricle circulation, neonatal heart transplantation, or termination of pregnancy. Limited data demonstrated a 15-year survival of 39% in patients who received palliative surgery with 64% of deaths occurring at the time of the first surgery.[1] A subset of fetuses with aortic stenosis (AS) have a normal left ventricular size rather than hypoplasia on midgestation echocardiography, but will ultimately develop HLHS at birth. This suggests that the outflow tract obstruction is a potential precursor to HLHS. In utero aortic valvuloplasty, therefore, has the potential to lessen the severity of or prevent progression to HLHS. This study sought to determine features on prenatal echocardiogram that identify appropriate candidates.

OBJECTIVES

To identify the midgestation echocardiographic features that predict progression of fetal AS to HLHS.

METHODS

Retrospective study at a single US center from 1992 to 2004.

Patients

43 fetuses diagnosed at <30 weeks' gestation with predominantly valvular AS and a left ventricular diastolic length above the lower limit of normal. 23 live-born fetuses were followed. Select exclusion criteria: additional major cardiac defects, any fetal intervention.

Intervention

Review of anatomic and physiologic measurements on prenatal echocardiograms were performed by investigator blinded to outcomes.

Outcomes

Primary outcome was development of HLHS warranting stage I neonatal palliative procedure (Norwood).

KEY RESULTS

- Of 23 live-born neonates, 17 progressed to HLHS and 6 had biventricular circulation. There were 17 terminated pregnancies, 1 fetal demise, and 2 lost to follow-up.
- Physiologic features were predictive of progression to HLHS: retrograde flow in the transverse aortic arch was present in 100%, left-to-right flow across the foramen ovale in 88%, monophasic mitral valve inflow in 91%, and moderate-to-severe left ventricular dysfunction in 94%. Those with biventricular circulation had none of these features.
- In contrast, no anatomic fetal echocardiogram findings reliably predicted progression to HLHS.

STUDY CONCLUSIONS

Specific physiologic findings on fetal echocardiogram at the time of diagnosis of AS predicted progression to HLHS.

COMMENTARY

This study helped determine which fetuses may benefit from aortic valvuloplasty, which has the potential to transform HLHS from a condition with poor prognosis to a preventable one. In support of these findings, a subsequent center reported that 30% of live-born neonates who underwent successful in utero aortic valvuloplasty were born with biventricular circulation.[2] However, nearly 10% of fetuses with successful valvuloplasty had fetal demise, indicating that the procedure does carry a high risk. Additionally, all neonates who were born with biventricular circulation after successful valvuloplasty required further postnatal interventions. Follow-up data are needed to determine if in utero valvuloplasty improves long-term survival of patients with HLHS.

Question

Is there a way to predict midgestation which fetuses with AS will develop HLHS?

Answer

Yes, 4 physiologic measurements on echocardiogram at the time of diagnosis of fetal AS are predictive of ultimate progression to HLHS: flow reversal in the transverse aortic arch, left-to-right flow across the foramen ovale, monophasic mitral valve inflow, and moderate-to-severe left ventricular dysfunction.

References

1. Mahle WT, Spray TL, Wernovsky G, et al. Survival after reconstructive surgery for hypoplastic left heart syndrome: A 15-year experience from a single institution. *Circulation.* 2000;102 (19 Suppl 3): III136–III141.
2. McElhinney DB, Marshall AC, Wilkins-Haug LE, et al. Predictors of technical success and postnatal biventricular outcome after in utero aortic valvuloplasty for aortic stenosis with evolving hypoplastic left heart syndrome. *Circulation.* 2009;120(15):1482–1490.

IMPACT OF WEIGHT ON OUTCOMES IN REPAIR OF CONGENITAL HEART DEFECTS

CHAPTER 9

Laura Flannery ■ Manuella Lahoud-Rahme

Results of 102 Cases of Complete Repair of Congenital Heart Defects in Patients Weighing 700 to 2500 Grams

Reddy VM, McElhinney DB, Sagrado T, et al. *J Thorac Cardiovasc Surg.* 1999; 117(2):324–331

BACKGROUND

Infants with congenital heart disease (CHD) are nearly twice as likely to be low birth weight (LBW) as infants without CHD.[1] Previous studies suggested that LBW infants have increased risk of poor outcomes from corrective surgical repair, likely due to the effects of cardiopulmonary bypass and associated intracranial bleeding. Consequently, definitive surgical intervention was often delayed, leading to potential heart failure, cardiogenic shock, and death. This study aimed to elucidate if weight or age was correlated with outcomes for infants who undergo CHD repair.

OBJECTIVES

To determine early and late outcomes of CHD repair in LBW infants.

METHODS

Retrospective record review at 1 US center from 1990 to 1997 with cross-sectional follow-up in 1997.

Patients

102 LBW infants (600 to 2,500 g) who underwent primary complete repair of CHD. 65% were preterm; all weighed <2,500 g at the time of repair. Median age at surgery was 16 days (range 1 to 137). Select exclusion criterion: isolated patent ductus arteriosus.

Intervention

Variables assessed included birth weight, gestational age, weight and age at the time of operation, preoperative morbidity, diagnosis, lesion complexity, and cardiopulmonary bypass time. Median follow-up was 30 months.

Outcomes

Primary outcomes were perioperative mortality (<30 days), late survival, and need for reintervention. Secondary outcomes included preoperative morbidity, growth, and neurologic abnormalities.

KEY RESULTS

- 10 patients (9.8%) died perioperatively. Longer cardiopulmonary bypass time (251 ± 157 vs. 147 ± 49 minutes, $p < 0.001$) and longer aortic cross-clamp time (102 ± 52 vs. 78 ± 29 minutes, $p = 0.01$) correlated with early death, but weight and age did not.
- 84 patients (82%) survived >1 year. Longer cardiopulmonary bypass time was the only variable that correlated with worse late survival ($p = 0.001$).
- Freedom from reintervention was 91% at >1 year with no associated risk factors.
- Patients with high preoperative morbidity (e.g., persistent failure to thrive, prolonged intubation) were significantly older at the time of operation than patients without complications (41 ± 32 days vs. 22 ± 25 days, $p = 0.005$).
- At follow-up, none of the surviving patients had clinical evidence of postoperative neurologic abnormalities. Their growth approximated the average growth curves for LBW infants without CHD.

STUDY CONCLUSIONS

Gestational age, birth weight, and weight and age at operation were not correlated with perioperative mortality, late survival, or freedom from reintervention. Older patients had a higher morbidity prior to surgery. Together, this supported early repair for CHD.

COMMENTARY

Despite the small size, this study showed that no preoperative patient characteristics were significantly associated with adverse outcomes after surgical repair. Rather, longer cardiopulmonary bypass duration was the only variable with a consistent correlation with both early and late mortality, which may be confounded by lesion complexity requiring longer repair. This study also demonstrated that infants who were older at the time of repair had more significant preoperative morbidity, possibly related to consequences of prolonged cardiovascular compromise. An earlier surgical intervention may help to mitigate these morbidities. For this reason, more than a decade after this study, cardiac surgeons tend to operate on LBW infants at a younger age, although this remains institution specific.

Question

Is there a benefit to delaying repair of CHD in LBW infants?

Answer

No. Outcomes do not differ with respect to gestational age, birth weight, age, or weight at the time of surgery. Delaying repair does not confer any benefit and is associated with higher preoperative morbidity.

Reference

1. Kramer HH, Trampisch HJ, Rammos S, et al. Birth weight of children with congenital heart disease. *Eur J Pediatr.* 1990;149(11):752–757.

CHAPTER 10

SUDDEN DEATH IN YOUNG ATHLETES

Laura Flannery ■ Manuella Lahoud-Rahme

Sudden Death in Young Competitive Athletes. Clinical, Demographic, and Pathological Profiles

Maron BJ, Shirani J, Poliac LC, et al. *JAMA*. 1996;276(3):199–204

BACKGROUND

Sudden death in young athletes is rare but tragic, with an estimated 10 to 25 deaths annually in the US.[1] Consequently, there has been debate regarding the effectiveness of efforts to identify at-risk athletes through preparticipation screening. This study sought to add to limited evidence to inform best practices.

OBJECTIVES

To develop a clinical, demographic, and pathologic profile of young athletes with sudden death.

METHODS

Systematic analysis of case series of sudden deaths of young athletes identified from school reports, news media, and national registries from 1985 to 1995.

Patients

158 individuals ages 12 to 40 years in competitive sports programs who suffered sudden death. Select exclusion criteria: evidence of drug use on postmortem toxicology, inadequate autopsy records.

Intervention

Clinical information and circumstances surrounding sudden death were ascertained through interviews with family members, witnesses, and coaches and through analyses of postmortem anatomic, microscopic, and toxicologic data.

Outcomes

Primary outcomes were characteristics of athletes and probably causes of death.

KEY RESULTS

- 83% (134/158) of athletes had cardiovascular disease as the cause of death. The majority had structural defects: 36% (48) had hypertrophic cardiomyopathy, 10% (14) possible hypertrophic cardiomyopathy, and 13% (17) aberrant coronary arteries.
- 90% (120/134) of these athletes were male, and 68% (92/134) played basketball or football.
- Only 18% (24/134) had cardiovascular symptoms in the 36 months preceding death (e.g., chest pain, exertional dyspnea, syncope, and presyncope).

- 97% (130/134) of those with a cardiac etiology for sudden death had a preparticipation medical evaluation: only 15% (19) had symptoms or examination findings which raised suspicion of cardiovascular disease and only 6% (8) had the correct cardiovascular diagnosis made.

STUDY CONCLUSIONS

The majority of sudden death in athletes had a cardiovascular cause, most commonly hypertrophic cardiomyopathy. Very few athletes had preceding symptoms or signs that indicated underlying pathology; preparticipation medical evaluations did not reveal these cardiovascular diseases in the vast majority.

COMMENTARY

It is remarkable that the majority of athletes had a preparticipation medical evaluation, but that so few evaluations revealed pathology. Of note, this study did not account for those with cardiac anomalies identified by screening who subsequently removed themselves from competitive athletics, thereby preventing a possible death. However, no studies to date have linked preparticipation screening with lower mortality rates, including studies performed after implementation of a regional preparticipation screening program in Italy that included electrocardiography.[2] Currently, the American Heart Association/American College of Cardiology recommends a 12-point preparticipation cardiovascular screening which incorporates elements of personal history, family history, and physical examination (Table 10.1).[3]

Question

What causes sudden death in young competitive athletes, and can medical evaluation detect these causes prior to death?

Answer

The majority of deaths are caused by cardiovascular pathology, with hypertrophic cardiomyopathy being the most common; unfortunately, the vast majority of these defects are not detected in preparticipation medical screening.

References

1. Liberthson RR. Sudden death from cardiac causes in children and young adults. *N Engl J Med.* 1996; 334(16):1039–1044.
2. Maron BJ, Hass TS, Doerer JJ, et al. Comparison of U.S. and Italian experiences with sudden cardiac deaths in young competitive athletes and implications for preparticipation screening strategies. *Am J Cardiol.* 2009;104(2):276–280.
3. Maron BJ, Thompson PD, Ackerman MJ, et al. Recommendations and considerations related to preparticipation screening for cardiovascular abnormalities in competitive athletes: 2007 update: A scientific statement from the American Heart Association Council on Nutrition, Physical Activity, and Metabolism: Endorsed by the American College of Cardiology Foundation. *Circulation.* 2007;115:1643–1655.

Table 10.1 The 12-Element American Heart Association Recommendations for Preparticipation Cardiovascular Screening of Competitive Athletes

Personal History
    Exertional chest pain or discomfort
    Unexplained syncope or near-syncope
    History of heart murmur
    Elevated blood pressure

Family History
    Unexpected sudden death under the age of 50 in >1 relative
    Disability from heart disease under the age of 50 in >1 relative
    History of cardiomyopathies, long QT syndrome, channelopathies, Marfan syndrome, or
        arrhythmias

Physical Examination
    Heart murmur
    Femoral pulses
    Physical stigmata of Marfan syndrome
    Blood pressure, preferably in both arms

CRITICAL CARE

11. Early Antibiotics in Pediatric Sepsis
12. Interruption of Sedation for Early Extubation
13. Bundled Care for Reduction of Central Line Infections
14. High-Flow Nasal Cannula for Bronchiolitis
15. Bystander CPR in Pediatric Out-of-Hospital Cardiac Arrest
16. Restrictive Protocol for Blood Transfusions
17. Low Tidal Volume Ventilation in Acute Respiratory Distress Syndrome
18. Early Fluid Resuscitation in Septic Shock

EARLY ANTIBIOTICS IN PEDIATRIC SEPSIS

CHAPTER 11

Carolyn Murphy Boscia ■ Brian M. Cummings

Delayed Antimicrobial Therapy Increases Mortality and Organ Dysfunction Duration in Pediatric Sepsis
Weiss SL, Fitzgerald JC, Balamuth F, et al. *Crit Care Med.* 2014;42(11):2409–2417

BACKGROUND

Sepsis carries a 10% to 20% mortality rate in children who require pediatric intensive care unit (PICU) admission.[1] In adult sepsis, timely administration of appropriate antibiotics is known to reduce mortality; the Surviving Sepsis Campaign advocates for administration of effective antibiotics within the first hour after recognition of severe sepsis or septic shock. This study investigated whether early antibiotic administration was similarly impactful in pediatric sepsis.

OBJECTIVES

To assess whether delayed initiation of antibiotic therapy is associated with increased mortality and prolonged organ dysfunction in PICU patients with severe sepsis or septic shock.

METHODS

Retrospective, observational study in a single academic PICU from 2012 to 2013.

Patients

130 patients ages 1 to 15 years with sepsis or septic shock requiring PICU treatment. Select exclusion criterion: sepsis diagnosed prior to transfer from an outside facility.

Intervention

Early administration of antibiotics after initial recognition of sepsis. Recognition was defined as the time of ED triage or first sepsis-related intervention (e.g., ordering antibiotics or collecting blood culture) for non-ED patients.

Outcomes

Primary outcome was PICU mortality. Secondary outcomes were PICU length of stay following sepsis recognition, and number of days during which patients were stable (no vasopressors, ventilatory support, or organ failure).

KEY RESULTS

- There was increased mortality in children whose first antibiotics were given >3 hours after sepsis recognition as compared to those who received antibiotics within 1 hour (23% vs. 8%).

- Greater than 3-hour delay to first antibiotics was an independent risk factor for mortality (OR 3.83, 95% CI 1.06–13.82), and resulted in median increase of 4 days with organ failure per patient ($p = 0.04$).
- Mortality did not differ between patients who received appropriate vs. inappropriate initial antimicrobial therapy ($p = 0.76$); of note most initial therapy was appropriate.
- Patients who were treated with an institutional clinical pathway for sepsis had a shorter average time to initial antibiotic administration, 101 minutes vs. 181 minutes ($p < 0.01$).

STUDY CONCLUSIONS

Delayed antimicrobial therapy in severe sepsis and septic shock was an independent risk factor for mortality in PICU patients, reaching statistical significance in this study at the 3-hour mark.

COMMENTARY

This study was the first to show a mortality benefit to early antimicrobial therapy in children with sepsis. A trend toward improved mortality at time points earlier than 3 hours failed to reach statistical significance due to small sample size and relatively low overall mortality rate in pediatric sepsis. Larger studies are needed to prove the applicability in pediatrics of the Surviving Sepsis Campaign's 1-hour benchmark for antibiotic administration.[2] Importantly, this study demonstrated that an institutional sepsis protocol can dramatically improve time to antibiotic administration and sepsis treatment across a wide variety of settings.

Question

Does time to antibiotic administration influence mortality outcomes in pediatric sepsis?

Answer

Yes, administration of first antibiotics within 3 hours reduces mortality and burden of organ failure in children with sepsis; further studies are needed to determine whether the 1-hour window that has proven significant in the adult population is associated with definitive benefit in children.

References

1. Kutko MC, Calarco MP, Flaherty MB, et al. Mortality rates in pediatric septic shock with and without multiple organ system failure. *Pediatr Crit Care Med.* 2003;4(3):333–337.
2. Dellinger RP, Levy MM, Rhodes A, et al. Surviving sepsis campaign: International guidelines for management of severe sepsis and septic shock: 2012. *Crit Care Med.* 2013;41(2):580–637.

CHAPTER 12
INTERRUPTION OF SEDATION FOR EARLY EXTUBATION

Carolyn Murphy Boscia ■ Brian M. Cummings

Randomized Controlled Trial of Daily Interruption of Sedatives in Critically Ill Children
Verlaat CW, Heesen GP, Vet NJ, et al. *Paediatr Anaesth.* 2014;24(2):151–156

BACKGROUND
Continuous sedation during intubation in the pediatric intensive care unit (PICU) allows for adequate pain control and anxiolysis, but carries risks of tolerance, withdrawal, and prolonged recovery. Daily sedation breaks shorten intubation duration and ICU length of stay in adults; this study assessed efficacy of sedation interruption in the PICU setting.

OBJECTIVES
To assess whether daily sedation breaks in PICU patients are feasible and to measure their impact on sedative dosing.

METHODS
Open-label randomized controlled trial in a 13-bed PICU in the Netherlands from 2004 to 2006.

Patients
30 patients ages 0 to 12 years, intubated >24 hours, and requiring continued mechanical ventilation for >48 hours. Select exclusion criteria: limited ability to assess sedation (e.g., neurologic compromise, neuromuscular blockade), second indication for sedation (e.g., pulmonary hypertension), upper airway pathology, life expectancy <1 month.

Intervention
Daily interruption of sedatives (morphine and midazolam) compared with routine staff-directed sedation administration. Assessments were performed with COMFORT-B observational scale of distress level. Agitation was treated by bolusing sedatives and increasing (or restarting) the continuous infusion.

Outcomes
Primary outcomes were number of boluses and cumulative doses of each sedative during the first 3 days, and number of adverse incidents or near incidents (e.g., unintended extubation). Secondary outcomes were duration of mechanical ventilation and PICU admission, and changes in COMFORT-B score.

KEY RESULTS
- Overall sedative use during the first 3 days decreased more dramatically in the intervention vs. control group (80% vs. 25% for midazolam, $p = 0.007$; 75% vs. 50% for morphine, $p = 0.02$).

- The intervention group had shorter average intubation (4 vs. 9 days, $p = 0.03$) and PICU stay (6 vs. 10 days, $p = 0.01$) compared to the control group.
- Bolus dose requirements were equivalent between groups ($p = 0.98$).
- There were no unintended extubations and no increase in overall adverse events in the intervention group.

STUDY CONCLUSIONS

Daily interruption of sedation in intubated children decreased use of sedatives, shortened duration of intubation and ICU length of stay, and was feasible.

COMMENTARY

This study was unblinded, and was partially confounded by variability in clinical attention, with intervention patients receiving 18 daily sedation assessments and control patients receiving only 5. Nonetheless, it showed remarkable efficacy. An ongoing multicenter study in the Netherlands may provide more robust data and establish safety parameters, which this study was underpowered to do. Nursing-driven sedation weaning protocols show similar efficacy to sedation interruption in adult ICUs, but a recent pediatric study showed no benefit.[1,2] Since interrupted sedation appears to be the more effective strategy in children, more data are needed regarding its emotional impact. In adults, shortening sedation duration decreases post-traumatic stress disorder symptoms; however, in children, the experience of being awake while intubated might cause added trauma, which could outweigh benefits of reduced total sedation.[3]

Question

Does daily interruption of sedation improve outcomes in intubated children?

Answer

Yes; daily sedation breaks decrease sedative use and shorten duration of intubation and PICU length of stay.

References

1. Mehta S, Burry L, Cook D, et al. Daily sedation interruption in mechanically ventilated critically ill patients cared for with a sedation protocol: A randomized controlled trial. *JAMA*. 2012;308(19):1985–1992.
2. Curley MA, Wypij D, Watson RS, et al. Protocolized sedation vs usual care in pediatric patients mechanically ventilated for acute respiratory failure: A randomized clinical trial. *JAMA*. 2015;313(4):379–389.
3. Wade DM, Howell DC, Weinman JA, et al. Investigating risk factors for psychological morbidity three months after intensive care: A prospective cohort study. *Crit Care*. 2012;16(5):R192.

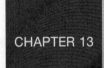

| CHAPTER 13 | BUNDLED CARE FOR REDUCTION OF CENTRAL LINE INFECTIONS |

Carolyn Murphy Boscia ■ Brian M. Cummings

Reducing PICU Central Line-Associated Bloodstream Infections: 3-Year Results
Miller MR, Niedner MF, Huskins WC, et al. *Pediatrics*. 2011;128(5):e1077–e1083

BACKGROUND

Each central line-associated bloodstream infection (CLABSI) in a child prolongs hospitalization by an average of 19 days, and adds approximately $56,000 to the costs of care.[1] Standardized care bundles can reduce CLABSI incidence in adult patients by about 66%; most of that improvement comes from safer line-insertion practices.[2] Since children have fewer central venous catheters (CVCs) placed, a greater proportion of their infection risk occurs during line maintenance. An initial pediatric study demonstrated a nearly 50% reduction in CLABSIs over 1 year using insertion and maintenance care bundles.[3] This follow-up study evaluated the sustainability of those improvements.

OBJECTIVES

To assess durability of improvement in CLABSI rates after implementation of standardized line-care practices, and to evaluate additional benefit from use of chlorhexidine scrubs and sponges.

METHODS

Interrupted time-series study in 29 pediatric intensive care units (PICUs) from 2006 to 2009, using preintervention historical control data from 2004 to 2006.

Patients

Children who required CVCs with total of 501,911 central line days during a 3-year period of postintervention observation.

Intervention

Implementation of care bundles for insertion (prepackaged kits, checklists, and insertion training) and maintenance (standardized dressing changes and daily assessment for discontinuation) of CVCs. Nested in the study was an 18-month nonrandomized evaluation of chlorhexidine-impregnated sponges and scrubs.

Outcomes

Primary outcome was the trend in monthly PICU CLABSI rate. Secondary outcome was the difference in CLABSI rates between bundle-only sites and bundle-plus-chlorhexidine sites. CLABSI definition was narrowed in 2008, requiring 2 positive blood culture results if organism was considered common skin contaminant.

KEY RESULTS

- There was a 56% decrease in average PICU CLABSI rate over the 3-year period, from 5.2/1,000 line-days (95% CI 4.4–6.2) to 2.3/1,000 line-days (95% CI 1.9–2.9).
- There was an 11% monthly decrease in CLABSI rate during implementation phase (95% CI 3–18).
- After the change in definition, CLABSI rate decreased by 15% over 1 month.
- The intervention cost $75,000 and saved $350,000 in CLABSI-related expenses per institution annually.
- Adding chlorhexidine products to the care bundles did not further decrease infection rates.

STUDY CONCLUSIONS

Consistent use of CVC care bundles in the PICU achieved significant and sustained decrease in the rate of CLABSI.

COMMENTARY

Reduction of healthcare-associated infections is a critical quality and safety priority and an increasingly important external regulatory mandate. This study demonstrated that simple checklists significantly reduce pediatric CLABSIs. Of note, the midstudy narrowing of the CLABSI definition quickly dropped the incidence by 15%; however, even when this change is discounted from the overall effect size of 56%, there remains an impressive 41% true reduction in CLABSIs over 3 years. This study resulted in the adoption of CLABSI prevention bundles as standard of care in pediatrics.

Question

Do standardized insertion and maintenance bundles for CVC care in the PICU result in a meaningful decrease in rates of line infection?

Answer

Yes; these protocols, along with staff training, are a cost-effective way to achieve sustained and significant reduction in CLABSI rates.

References

1. Goudie A, Dynan L, Brady PW, et al. Attributable cost and length of stay for central line-associated bloodstream infections. *Pediatrics.* 2014;133(6):e1525–e1532.
2. Pronovost P, Needham D, Berenholtz S, et al. An intervention to decrease catheter-related bloodstream infections in the ICU. *N Engl J Med.* 2006;355(26):2725–2732.
3. Miller MR, Griswold M, Harris JM II, et al. Decreasing PICU catheter-associated bloodstream infections: NACHRI's quality transformation efforts. *Pediatrics.* 2010;125(2):206–213.

CHAPTER 14

HIGH-FLOW NASAL CANNULA FOR BRONCHIOLITIS

Carolyn Murphy Boscia ■ Brian M. Cummings

High-Flow Nasal Cannulae Therapy in Infants With Bronchiolitis
McKiernan C, Chua LC, Visintainer PF, et al. *J Pediatr.* 2010;156(4):634–638

BACKGROUND

Bronchiolitis accounts for 16% of hospitalizations in US children under the age of 2 years, and over $500 million annually in healthcare spending.[1] There is currently no targeted treatment; severely ill children require intubation, putting them at risk for pneumonia and prolonged hospitalization. Continuous positive airway pressure (CPAP) is effective, but is rarely tolerated by young children. High-flow nasal cannula (HFNC), which delivers oxygen with a small amount of positive airway pressure, is better tolerated and is a well-established mode of ventilation in neonates. This was the first study examining the use of HFNC in infants with bronchiolitis.

OBJECTIVES

To determine whether HFNC therapy decreases intubation rates among infants with bronchiolitis admitted to the pediatric intensive care unit (PICU).

METHODS

Retrospective chart review in a single US PICU from 2005 to 2007.

Patients

115 children ages <24 months admitted to the PICU with diagnosis of bronchiolitis, respiratory distress, or respiratory failure. Select exclusion criterion: other respiratory diagnosis (e.g., reactive airway disease, pneumonia).

Intervention

Use of HFNC oxygen as the first-line noninvasive ventilatory strategy, as compared to the use of multiple modalities including conventional nasal cannula, nonrebreather masks, and nasal CPAP during the previous year.

Outcomes

Primary outcome was intubation rate before and after introduction of HFNC. Secondary outcomes were changes in respiratory parameters and intubation rates among subgroups stratified by age, weight, gestational age, and respiratory syncytial virus (RSV) status.

KEY RESULTS

- 87.9% (51/58) of post-intervention patients received initial respiratory support with HFNC, without any adverse events.

- Intubation rates decreased from 23% (13/57) to 9% (5/58) with the switch to HFNC ($p = 0.043$).
- HFNC implementation resulted in a 14% absolute and 68% RR reduction in the need for intubation, with a number needed to treat (NNT) of 7.
- Within the first hour of treatment, infants receiving HFNC had decreased respiratory rates by 12 additional breaths per minute as compared to those receiving other modalities ($p < 0.001$). Unimproved respiratory rate after 1 hour on HFNC was predictive of eventual intubation ($p < 0.03$).
- Median PICU length of stay decreased from 6 to 4 days after HFNC introduction ($p = 0.058$).

STUDY CONCLUSIONS

HFNC oxygen therapy decreased the need for intubation among infants with bronchiolitis in the PICU, without significant adverse effects.

COMMENTARY

This study demonstrated substantial improvement in outcomes with HFNC therapy. Lack of randomization and blinding left it vulnerable to observer-expectancy bias: if providers expected HFNC to be effective, it may have influenced their subjective decisions regarding intubation. However, the effect size was too large to attribute to bias alone. Moreover, the HFNC cohort's higher average initial respiratory rate and higher rate of RSV positivity (69% vs. 51%) suggested that they may have been sicker on presentation, making their better outcomes even more significant. These findings prompted widespread adoption of HFNC for bronchiolitis treatment in the PICU. However, a recent Cochrane review found insufficient evidence to state whether HFNC is effective in this setting, and further research is needed to draw definitive conclusions.[2]

Question

Does HFNC therapy improve outcomes in infants with bronchiolitis admitted to the PICU?

Answer

Yes; HFNC reduced intubation rates in this study and was well tolerated, leading to shorter PICU length of stay and fewer treatment-related complications. Large-scale studies are needed to robustly demonstrate its effectiveness.

References

1. Hasegawa K, Tsugawa Y, Brown DF, et al. Trends in bronchiolitis hospitalizations in the United States, 2000–2009. *Pediatrics.* 2013;132(1):28–36.
2. Beggs S, Wong ZH, Kaul S, et al. High-flow nasal cannula therapy for infants with bronchiolitis. *Cochrane Database Syst Rev.* 2014;(1):CD009609.

CHAPTER 15

BYSTANDER CPR IN PEDIATRIC OUT-OF-HOSPITAL CARDIAC ARREST

Carolyn Murphy Boscia ■ Brian M. Cummings

Conventional and Chest-Compression-Only Cardiopulmonary Resuscitation by Bystanders for Children Who Have Out-of-Hospital Cardiac Arrests: A Prospective, Nationwide, Population-based Cohort Study

Kitamura T, Iwami T, Kawamura T, et al. *Lancet.* 2010;375(9723):1347–1354

BACKGROUND

Most children receive no bystander cardiopulmonary resuscitation (CPR) during out-of-hospital cardiac arrest.[1] Compression-only CPR (COCPR) without rescue breathing is more readily performed than conventional CPR due to simplicity and lack of hygiene concerns, with resultant improvement in overall survival and neurologic prognosis in adult studies. The American Heart Association (AHA) exclusively recommends bystander COCPR in adults.[2] Pediatric cardiac arrest is most often of respiratory etiology, and it was unclear if COCPR was as effective in this population.

OBJECTIVES

To assess whether bystander CPR affects outcomes in pediatric cardiac arrest, and to compare efficacy of COCPR vs. conventional CPR in events of both primary cardiac and noncardiac etiology.

METHODS

Prospective, observational cohort study in Japan from 2005 to 2007.

Patients

5,170 patients ages <17 years with out-of-hospital cardiac arrest. Select exclusion criteria: arrest occurred after arrival of trained personnel, no documentation of witnessed vs. unwitnessed arrest.

Intervention

Japanese fire departments did community-based CPR training during the years before the study, reaching 1.4 million citizens annually; there was no teaching of COCPR. Data collected included demographics, cardiac rhythm, type of CPR delivered, and patient outcomes.

Outcomes

Primary outcome was favorable neurologic status 1 month after cardiac arrest. Secondary outcomes were return of spontaneous circulation before hospital arrival and 1-month survival.

KEY RESULTS
- 3,675 events were non-cardiac in etiology and 1,495 were primary cardiac arrests.
- 1,551 patients received conventional CPR and 888 received COCPR.
- Performance of any CPR improved neurologic outcomes at 1 month as compared to no CPR (adjusted OR 2.59, 95% CI 1.81–3.71).
- In events of noncardiac etiology, conventional CPR increased favorable neurologic outcome (adjusted OR 5.54, 95% CI 2.52–16.99) and 1-month survival (adjusted OR 1.89, 95% CI 1.23–2.91) as compared to COCPR.
- In primary cardiac events, conventional CPR and COCPR achieved equivalent neurologic outcomes and survival.
- Children <1 year old had poor outcomes regardless of etiology or CPR type performed.

STUDY CONCLUSIONS
Bystander CPR reduced morbidity and mortality in pediatric out-of-hospital cardiac arrests. CPR and COCPR were equally effective in primary cardiac arrest, but conventional CPR was more effective in noncardiac events.

COMMENTARY

Children who received any bystander CPR had far better outcomes than children who received none. One might conclude that conventional CPR should still be taught for pediatric arrests, since most of them are of noncardiac etiology. However, the bystander population was not trained in COCPR, which may account for its underperformance. An adult study in which laypersons were well trained showed equivalent outcomes between COCPR and conventional CPR even in primary respiratory arrests.[2] Implementation of unified training in COCPR for patients of all ages might increase rates of bystander CPR initiation in children and improve resuscitation technique. This could narrow the margin of underperformance of COCPR in noncardiac arrests and achieve overall better survival, which is an area for future research.

Question
Does bystander CPR improve neurologic outcomes and survival in pediatric out-of-hospital cardiac arrest?

Answer
Yes, bystander CPR significantly reduces morbidity and mortality in pediatric cardiac arrest; conventional and compression-only CPR are equally effective in primary cardiac arrest, but more data are needed to determine which method optimizes population-level outcomes.

References
1. Atkins DL, Everson-Stewart S, Sears GK, et al. Epidemiology and outcomes from out-of-hospital cardiac arrest in children: The Resuscitation Outcome Consortium Epistry-Cardiac Arrest. *Circulation.* 2009; 119(11):1484–1491.
2. Bobrow BJ, Spaite DW, Berg RA, et al. Chest compression-only CPR by lay rescuers and survival from out-of-hospital cardiac arrest. *JAMA.* 2010;304(13):1447–1454.

CHAPTER 16

RESTRICTIVE PROTOCOL FOR BLOOD TRANSFUSIONS

Matthew G. Gartland ■ Brian M. Cummings

Transfusion Strategies for Patients in Pediatric Intensive Care Units
Lacroix J, Hébert PC, Hutchison JS, et al. *N Engl J Med.* 2007;356(16):1609–1619

BACKGROUND
As many as 50% of critically ill children in the pediatric intensive care unit (PICU) may receive a blood transfusion for anemia.[1] However, blood transfusions are an expensive and limited resource with potential adverse effects, and the optimal hemoglobin (Hb) threshold requiring transfusion is unknown. Adult ICU studies showed equivalency at lower Hb transfusion thresholds, with a landmark study demonstrating increased mortality with a liberal transfusion strategy, prompting this pediatric study.

OBJECTIVES
To determine if a restrictive transfusion strategy is as safe as a liberal strategy in critically ill children in regard to development of multiorgan dysfunction syndrome (MODS).

METHODS
Randomized controlled noninferiority trial in 19 PICUs in 4 countries from 2001 to 2005.

Patients
637 children ages 3 days to 14 years who had Hb <9.5 g/dL within 7 days after PICU admission. Select exclusion criteria: expected PICU stay <24 hours, hemodynamic instability, hemolytic anemia, prematurity, hypoxemia.

Intervention
Weight-based leukocyte-reduced red blood cell transfusions were administered targeting either a liberal threshold (Hb 9.5 g/dL) or a restrictive threshold (Hb 7 g/dL). Physicians could temporarily suspend the protocol if patients became unstable.

Outcomes
Primary outcome was the development of new or progressive MODS (concurrent dysfunction of >2 organ systems or worsening dysfunction of >1 organ). Secondary outcomes included incidence of transfusion reactions, infections, and length of stay.

KEY RESULTS
- 12% of patients in both arms had new or progressive MODS. Restrictive arm received 44% fewer transfusions, with 54% of patients receiving no transfusions as compared to only 2% in the liberal arm ($p < 0.001$).

- No significant difference was noted in nosocomial infections, mechanical ventilation, transfusion reactions, or length of stay.
- Protocol was temporarily suspended more frequently in the restrictive arm than in the liberal arm (39 vs. 20 patients, $p = 0.01$). More patients received transfusions during suspension in the restrictive arm (36 vs. 11 patients, $p < 0.001$) than in the liberal arm.

STUDY CONCLUSIONS

A restrictive transfusion threshold (Hb 7 g/dL) was noninferior to a liberal transfusion threshold (Hb 9.5 g/dL) and resulted in fewer transfusions in children in the PICU.

COMMENTARY

This study was difficult to perform but critically necessary to confirm noninferiority of a restrictive transfusion strategy in pediatrics given the adult evidence of harm. It was limited by nonblinded design that allowed for a physician to temporarily suspend the protocol; however, this was practically important for enrollment due to strong clinician perceptions that blood is physiologically beneficial. Even with these protocol deviations, children in the restrictive group still received fewer transfusions. A restrictive strategy is now the standard of care in the PICU for stable patients. It remains unknown whether more liberal blood transfusions benefit subpopulations given mixed outcomes in cardiac conditions and preterm infants.[2,3]

Question

Is a restrictive transfusion strategy equivalent to a liberal strategy among critically ill children?

Answer

Yes; in this multicenter trial, the occurrence of multiorgan dysfunction occurred at similar rates among children randomized to both liberal and restrictive transfusion protocols; those in whom a lower Hb of 7 was targeted were exposed to significantly fewer transfusions.

References

1. Morris KP, Nagvi N, Davies P, et al. A new formula for blood transfusion volume in the critically ill. *Arch Dis Child.* 2005;90(7):724–728.
2. Jonas RA, Wypij D, Roth SJ, et al. The influence of hemodilution on outcome after hypothermic cardiopulmonary bypass: Results of a randomized trial in infants. *J Thorac Cardiovasc Surg.* 2003;126(6):1765–1774.
3. Bell EF, Strauss RG, Widness JA, et al. Randomized trial of liberal versus restrictive guidelines for red blood cell transfusion in preterm infants. *Pediatrics.* 2005;115(6):1685–1691.

LOW TIDAL VOLUME VENTILATION IN ACUTE RESPIRATORY DISTRESS SYNDROME

Matthew G. Gartland ■ Brian M. Cummings

Ventilation With Lower Tidal Volumes as Compared With Traditional Tidal Volumes for Acute Lung Injury and the Acute Respiratory Distress Syndrome

The Acute Respiratory Distress Syndrome Network. *N Engl J Med*. 2000;342(18): 1301–1308

BACKGROUND

Acute respiratory distress syndrome (ARDS) and acute lung injury (ALI), now called mild ARDS, carry high mortality in adults and children. Traditional mechanical ventilation strategies to maximize oxygenation and achieve normal values of pH and partial pressure of CO_2 ($PaCO_2$) in ARDS used physiologic or larger tidal volumes (TVs). However, potential harms demonstrated in animal models included lung stretch injury (volutrauma) and barotrauma, possibly due to high positive pressures. Prior to this study, the impact of lung injury in human trials was inconclusive.

OBJECTIVES

To assess whether lower TV ventilation improves mortality in adults with ARDS.

METHODS

Randomized controlled trial at 10 US centers from 1996 to 1999.

Patients

861 patients ages 18 to 70 years with ARDS and ALI, defined as acute decrease in the ratio of partial pressure of arterial oxygen (PaO_2) to fraction of inspired oxygen (FiO_2) to <300, chest x-ray with bilateral infiltrates, and no evidence of left atrial hypertension. Select exclusion criterion: life expectancy <6 months.

Intervention

With volume-control mode, traditional group received ~12 mL/kg TV with plateau pressure <50 cm H_2O and low TV group received ~6 mL/kg with plateau pressures <30 cm H_2O.

Outcomes

Primary outcomes were death before discharge home and breathing without assistance, and ventilator-free days in first 28 days after intubation.

KEY RESULTS

- 432 patients received mean TV of 6.2 ± 0.8 mL and 429 patients received 11.8 ± 0.8 mL in their first 3 days of hospitalization ($p < 0.001$). Mean plateau pressures were 25 ± 6 and 33 ± 8 cm H_2O, respectively ($p < 0.001$).

- Mortality in the low TV group was 22% lower than in the traditional group (31% vs. 39.8%, $p = 0.007$).
- There were more ventilator-free days (12 vs. 10, $p = 0.007$) and days without organ failure (15 vs. 12, $p = 0.006$) in the low TV group than in the traditional group.
- Low TV group had higher $PaCO_2$ and lower pH, and required higher positive end-expiratory pressure (PEEP) and FiO_2 to maintain PaO_2.

STUDY CONCLUSIONS

Lower TV ventilation (6 mL/kg) decreased mortality and increased ventilator-free days compared to traditional TV ventilation (12 mL/kg) in adults with ARDS.

COMMENTARY

This study was terminated early due to the significant benefits from lower TV ventilation, even with the higher PEEP and FiO_2 requirements to maintain adequate oxygenation. Benefits are postulated to be related to reductions in volutrauma or reduced atelectasis and reexpansion injury with higher PEEP. The use of low TV ventilation targeting lower plateau pressures is supported by subsequent trials and is now standard of care for adults with ARDS.[1] Although not specifically evaluated in children, these findings were significant enough that lower TV ventilation has also become standard of care in pediatric ARDS, yet variability in practice remains.[2,3]

Question

Is lower TV ventilation (6 mL/kg) superior to traditional volume ventilation (12 mL/kg) in adults with ARDS?

Answer

Yes; lower TV results in reduced mortality and ventilator-free days, and has become standard of care. These findings have been extrapolated to care of children with ARDS.

References

1. Putensen C, Theuerkauf N, Zinserling J, et al. Meta-analysis: Ventilation strategies and outcomes of the acute respiratory distress syndrome and acute lung injury. *Ann Intern Med.* 2009;151(8):566–576.
2. Cornfield D. Acute respiratory distress syndrome in children: Physiology and management. *Curr Opin Pediatr.* 2013;25(3):338–343.
3. Santschi M, Randolph AG, Rimensberger PC, et al. Mechanical ventilation strategies in children with acute lung injury: A survey on stated practice pattern. *Pediatr Crit Care Med.* 2013;14(7):e332–e337.

CHAPTER 18	EARLY FLUID RESUSCITATION IN SEPTIC SHOCK

Matthew G. Gartland ■ Brian M. Cummings

Role of Early Fluid Resuscitation in Pediatric Septic Shock
Carcillo JA, Davis AL, Zaritsky A. *JAMA.* 1991;266(9):1242–1245

BACKGROUND
The management of septic shock in children is challenging as patients can exhibit signs of hypovolemic, cardiogenic, and distributive shock. Treatment of septic shock with volume resuscitation may improve oxygen delivery and support cardiac output but can also result in cardiogenic or noncardiogenic pulmonary edema, now known as acute respiratory distress syndrome (ARDS). This small study performed over 20 years ago was the first to examine the role of aggressive volume resuscitation in children with septic shock.

OBJECTIVES
To assess the impact of early aggressive fluid management on survival and complications in pediatric septic shock.

METHODS
Prospective, nonrandomized cohort study at a single US center from 1982 to 1989.

Patients
34 children ages 1 month to 16 years with shock (blood pressure <2 standard deviations below mean for age), poor perfusion, and positive blood or tissue culture who had placement of a pulmonary artery catheter within 6 hours of presentation. Select exclusion criteria: none.

Intervention
Patients were stratified into 3 groups based on the volume of crystalloid fluid received within the first hour of presentation to the emergency department: <20 mL/kg (group 1), 20 to 40 mL/kg (group 2), and >40 mL/kg (group 3). Volume status was reassessed at 6 hours.

Outcomes
Primary outcome was survival to hospital discharge. Secondary outcomes included development of ARDS, cardiogenic pulmonary edema, or persistent hypovolemia.

KEY RESULTS
- There was lower mortality among children who received more fluid: 57% (8/15) in group 1, 64% (7/11) in group 2, and 11% (1/9) in group 3 ($p = 0.039$).

- No increase was seen in noncardiogenic or cardiogenic pulmonary edema among children who received more IV fluid.
- All patients required vasopressor agents.
- 8 patients from groups 1 and 2 were persistently hypovolemic at 6 hours and all 8 died. Nonsurvivors across all groups received significantly less fluid at 1 hour than survivors (23 ± 18 mL/kg vs. 42 ± 28 mL/kg, $p < 0.05$), but received similar quantities at 6 hours.

STUDY CONCLUSIONS

Early, rapid, and aggressive fluid resuscitation (>40 mL/kg in first hour) in children with septic shock was associated with improved survival, and did not increase the incidence of pulmonary edema.

COMMENTARY

This study shaped the development of sepsis guidelines by the American College of Critical Care Medicine and Pediatric Advanced Life Support, offering a powerful intervention for a condition with high mortality. Study limitations included a small sample recruited over a long time period during which there were many other medical advancements, lack of acuity scoring, and inability to adjust for confounders (e.g., chronic disease). The recent FEAST trial conducted in East Africa suggested potential harm of this strategy in resource-poor settings. As that study population included patients who had late presentation to the hospital, malnutrition, and anemia with no access to intensive critical care services, generalizability is limited.[1] Therefore, rapid aggressive fluid resuscitation remains standard of care for treatment of pediatric septic shock, along with inotrope, vasopressor, and hydrocortisone therapy in refractory shock.[2]

Question

Do children with septic shock benefit from IV fluid administration?

Answer

Yes. In this small prospective cohort study, children receiving more than 40 mL/kg of crystalloid fluid within the first hour of presentation had decreased mortality without increased pulmonary edema.

References

1. Maitland K, Kiguli S, Opoka RO, et al. Mortality after fluid bolus in African children with severe infection. *N Engl J Med.* 2011;364(26):2483–2495.
2. Dellinger RP, Levy MM, Rhodes A, et al. Surviving sepsis campaign: International guidelines for management of severe sepsis and septic shock: 2012. *Crit Care Med.* 2013;41(2):580–637.

EMERGENCY MEDICINE

19. A Prediction Rule for Appendicitis
20. Need for CT Scan in Head Trauma
21. Utility of Lumbar Puncture in First Simple Febrile Seizure
22. Oral Ondansetron for Gastroenteritis
23. Oral Versus Intravenous Rehydration
24. Oral Dexamethasone for Mild Croup
25. Likelihood of Occult Pneumonia in Febrile Children
26. Ipratropium in Acute Asthma Management
27. Evaluation of the Febrile Infant

| CHAPTER 19 | # A PREDICTION RULE FOR APPENDICITIS |

Thomas F. Heyne ■ Lauren Allister

Validation and Refinement of a Prediction Rule to Identify Children at Low Risk for Acute Appendicitis

Kharbanda AB, Dudley NC, Bajaj L, et al. *Arch Pediatr Adolesc Med.* 2012;166(8):738–744

BACKGROUND

Appendicitis is the most common pediatric surgical emergency, although fewer than 1% of children presenting with acute abdominal pain have appendicitis.[1] Concern over morbidity from missed diagnoses may lead to unnecessary surgery or CT-related radiation exposure. In 2005, a clinical prediction rule was devised to identify children at low risk for appendicitis. It showed an NPV of 98% when none of the following features were present: absolute neutrophil count (ANC) $\leq 6.75 \times 10^3/\mu L$, absence of nausea, and absence of maximal tenderness in the right lower quadrant (RLQ).[2] This study was conducted to further refine this rule.

OBJECTIVES

To validate and refine a prediction rule that identifies children with acute abdominal pain at low risk for appendicitis.

METHODS

Prospective, cross-sectional study in 9 US pediatric emergency departments (ED) from 2009 to 2010.

Patients

2,625 children ages 3 to 18 years with <96 hours of abdominal pain undergoing evaluation for appendicitis. Select exclusion criteria: pregnancy, chronic abdominal pain, prior abdominal surgery, sickle cell anemia, recent abdominal trauma.

Intervention

Standard history and physical examinations were performed. Decisions regarding imaging, consults, and disposition were at physicians' discretion. Relevant records were reviewed and phone calls were conducted within 2 weeks to document final disposition.

Outcomes

Primary outcome was performance of the clinical prediction rule to identify children at low risk for appendicitis, based on pathology or operative report.

KEY RESULTS

- 38.8% (1,018/2,625) of enrolled patients had appendicitis (95% CI 36.9–40.7).
- The original rule had an NPV of 92.7%, and misclassified 4.5% of patients (95% CI 3.4–6.1) with appendicitis as low risk.
- A refined rule defined low risk as ANC $\leq 6.75 \times 10^3/\mu L$ and either no maximal tenderness in the RLQ or no abdominal pain with walking, jumping, or coughing. Sensitivity was 98.1% (95% CI 97–98.9), specificity was 23.7% (95% CI 21.7–25.9), and NPV was 95.3% (95% CI 92.3–97).
- Of 400 patients identified as low risk, 8 (2%) underwent a negative appendectomy and 180 (45%) received a CT scan. 19/400 (4.8%) had appendicitis (falsely classified as low risk).

STUDY CONCLUSIONS

A refined prediction rule (ANC $\leq 6.75 \times 10^3/\mu L$, and either no maximal tenderness at RLQ, or no pain with walking, jumping, or coughing) helped identify children at low risk of appendicitis.

COMMENTARY

This study attempted to reduce reliance on diagnostic imaging and improve efficiency in diagnosing appendicitis. While no single clinical prediction rule has become standard practice, this study provides a validated and practical approach to identify children in whom watchful waiting or ultrasound may be a reasonable alternative. Study limitations include enrollment exclusively in pediatric EDs and a high rate of appendicitis (>30%). The utilization of new inflammatory markers (e.g., procalcitonin), alone and in concert with other variables, may further help to refine diagnostic algorithms for appendicitis in future studies without reliance on imaging at all.

Question

Do all children need CT imaging as part of the evaluation for suspected appendicitis?

Answer

No. When the ANC is $\leq 6.75 \times 10^3/\mu L$, and children have either no maximal tenderness at the RLQ, or RLQ tenderness but no pain with walking, jumping, or coughing, there is a low risk of acute appendicitis and expectant management is appropriate.

References

1. Scholer SJ, Pituch K, Orr DP, et al. Clinical outcomes of children with acute abdominal pain. *Pediatrics.* 1996;98:680–685.
2. Kharbanda AB, Taylor GA, Fishman SJ, et al. A clinical decision rule to identify children at low risk for appendicitis. *Pediatrics.* 2005;116(3):709–716.

CHAPTER 20

NEED FOR CT SCAN IN HEAD TRAUMA

Thomas F. Heyne ■ Lauren Allister

Identification of Children at Very Low Risk of Clinically-Important Brain Injuries After Head Trauma: A Prospective Cohort Study

Kuppermann N, Holmes JF, Dayan PS, et al. *Lancet.* 2009;374(9696):1160–1170

BACKGROUND

Head trauma in children accounts for over 600,000 emergency department (ED) visits annually: approximately 2% of cases represent clinically important traumatic brain injury (ciTBI), defined as injury requiring acute intervention.[1,2] Head CT was previously used especially in preverbal children unable to provide a history, but the ionizing radiation poses a long-term malignancy risk. Prior to this study, clinical prediction rules existed to identify adult patients most likely to benefit from head CT, but no such rules existed for children.

OBJECTIVES

To derive and validate age-specific clinical decision rules to identify children with blunt head trauma who are at very low risk for ciTBI.

METHODS

Prospective cohort derivation and validation study in 25 US EDs within the Pediatric Emergency Care Applied Research Network (PECARN) from 2004 to 2006.

Patients

42,412 children ages <18 years presenting <24 hours after head trauma with Glasgow Coma Scale (GCS) scores of 14 to 15. Select exclusion criteria: low-risk injury mechanisms, penetrating trauma, pre-existing neurologic conditions, bleeding disorder, or ventricular shunt.

Intervention

Data from history, physical examination, imaging (if obtained), and outcomes were reviewed, and age-specific clinical decision rules were derived with subsequent validation in a smaller cohort. Clinical decision making was at physicians' discretion. Follow-up calls were conducted at 7 and 90 days.

Outcomes

Primary outcome was presence of ciTBI (TBI on CT associated with at least one of the following: death from TBI, need for neurosurgery, hospital admission ≥2 nights, or intubation >24 hours).

KEY RESULTS

- 35.3% (n = 14,969) of children had CT scans. Of these, 5.2% (n = 780) had TBI, 0.9% (n = 376) had ciTBI, and 0.1% (n = 60) required neurosurgery.
- For children <2 years, the absence of 6 specific predictors (altered mental status [AMS], nonfrontal scalp hematoma, loss of consciousness [LOC] ≥5 seconds, severe mechanism of injury, palpable skull fracture, or not acting normally) yielded an NPV for ciTBI of 100% (1,175/1,175, 95% CI 99.7–100.0).
- For children ≥2 years, the absence of 6 different predictors (AMS, LOC, vomiting, severe injury mechanism, signs of basilar skull fracture, or severe headache) yielded an NPV for ciTBI of 99.95% (3,798/3,800, 95% CI 99.8–99.9).

STUDY CONCLUSIONS

The clinical decision rules derived and validated in this study were sensitive in identifying children with blunt head trauma at low risk for ciTBI, who did not require CT imaging.

COMMENTARY

This landmark study developed rules to help avoid unnecessary CT scans, particularly in the younger children at greatest risk of malignancy from radiation exposure. The major study limitation was that not every child underwent CT imaging; however, follow-up was used as a reasonable surrogate to rule out the presence of ciTBI. These rules are assistive only, and parental preference and clinician experience must be considered, particularly in children with multiple injuries, worsening symptoms, or age <3 months.

Question

Are there predictive factors to identify children at low risk for significant traumatic brain injury after minor head trauma?

Answer

Yes, this study derived and validated age-specific prediction rules (reproduced below; Fig. 20.1) to identify patients unlikely to benefit from CT imaging.

References

1. Faul M, Xu L, Wald MM, et al. *Traumatic Brain Injury in the United States: Emergency Department Visits, Hospitalizations and Deaths 2002–2006.* Atlanta, GA: Centers for Disease Control and Prevention; National Center for Injury Prevention and Control; 2010.
2. Easter JS, Bakes K, Dhaliwal J, et al. Comparison of PECARN, CATCH, and CHALICE rules for children with minor head injury: A prospective cohort study. *Ann Emerg Med.* 2014;64(2):145–152, 152.e1–e5.

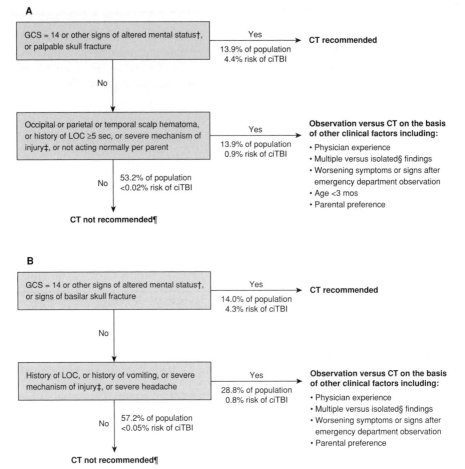

Figure 20.1 Suggested CT algorithm for **(A)** children <2 years old and **(B)** ≥2 years old with Glasgow Coma Scale (GCS) of 14-15 after head trauma. ciTBI=clinically-important traumatic brain injury. LOC=loss of consciousness.*

*Data are from the combined derivation and validation populations.

†Other signs of altered mental status: agitation, somnolence, repetitive questioning, or slow response to verbal communication.

‡Severe mechanism of injury: motor vehicle crash with patient ejection, death of another passenger, or rollover; pedestrian or bicyclist without helmet struck by a motorised vehicle; falls of more than 0.9 m (3 feet) (or more than 1.5 m [5 feet] for panel B); or head struck by a high-impact object.

§Patients with certain isolated findings (ie, with no other findings suggestive of traumatic brain injury), such as isolated LOC, isolated headache, isolated vomiting, and certain types of isolated scalp haematomas in infants older than 3 months, have a risk of ciTBI substantially lower than 1%.

¶Risk of ciTBI exceedingly low, generally lower than risk of CT-induced malignancies. Therefore, CT scans are not indicated for most patients in this group. (From Kuppermann N, Holmes JF, Dayan PS, et al. Identification of children at very low risk of clinically important brain injuries after head trauma: A prospective cohort study. *Lancet.* 2009;374(9696):1160–1170, Figure 3.)

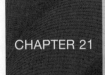

UTILITY OF LUMBAR
CHAPTER 21   PUNCTURE IN FIRST SIMPLE
FEBRILE SEIZURE

Thomas F. Heyne ■ Lauren Allister

Utility of Lumbar Puncture for First Simple Febrile Seizure Among Children 6 to 18 Months of Age

Kimia AA, Capraro AJ, Hummel D, et al. *Pediatrics*. 2009;123(1):6–12

BACKGROUND

In 1996, the American Academy of Pediatrics (AAP) issued practice parameters for managing infants with a first simple febrile seizure (FSFS) to assess for bacterial meningitis. These guidelines recommended lumbar puncture (LP) be strongly considered for infants 6 to 12 months of age and considered for children 12 to 18 months of age. As meningitis rates declined following the introduction of highly effective conjugate vaccines (for *Haemophilus influenzae b* and *Streptococcus pneumoniae*), this study sought to investigate the incidence of bacterial meningitis in young children with FSFS.

OBJECTIVES

To determine bacterial meningitis rates in otherwise healthy infants and young children with FSFS, and assess pediatric emergency department (ED) physician compliance with AAP guidelines for LP.

METHODS

Retrospective cohort study in a single US pediatric ED from 1995 to 2006.

Patients

704 children ages 6 to 18 months presenting within 12 hours of FSFS (≤15 minutes duration, no recurrence in 24 hours) who were otherwise well-appearing. Select exclusion criteria: prior seizure, chronic illness, trauma, irritability, lethargy.

Intervention

Medical record data were obtained regarding seizure characteristics, vaccine history, physical examination findings, LP attempts, cerebrospinal fluid (CSF) results, and subsequent outcome.

Outcomes

Primary outcome was meningitis rate defined by CSF growth of a pathogen, CSF pleocytosis (>7 white blood cells/mm^3) and positive blood culture, or positive CSF Gram stain. Secondary outcome was compliance with AAP recommendations (defined as any LP attempt including unsuccessful or refused).

KEY RESULTS
- No patients had bacterial meningitis: 0% (0/260) of CSF specimens grew any pathogens, 3.8% (10/260) grew a contaminant, and 3.8% (10/260) showed CSF pleocytosis without bacterial growth.
- 10% (68/704) of patients received antibiotics prior to LP, but none were subsequently found to have meningitis.
- LPs were attempted in 70% (131/188) of 6 to 12 month olds and 25% (129/516) of 12 to 18 month olds.

STUDY CONCLUSIONS
The rate of bacterial meningitis in this cohort of otherwise healthy children 6 to 18 months old presenting with FSFS was 0%. Provider compliance with the 1996 AAP guidelines was higher than in previous studies, but decreased over the study period, most notably in the 12- to 18-month age group.

COMMENTARY
This study established the low risk of bacterial meningitis in 6 to 18 month olds presenting with FSFS in the post-conjugate vaccine era. These findings informed the 2011 AAP FSFS guidelines recommending that LP only be performed in fully vaccinated children in this age group if there are concerning signs or symptoms.[1] Study limitations included a study population with a high vaccination rate (>90%). For patients <6 months of age who have not completed their primary vaccination series and in whom clinical clues for meningitis may be less apparent, as well as for older children who are ill appearing or have complex febrile seizures, LP must be considered on a case-by-case basis.

Question
Should LP be performed in otherwise healthy, well appearing 6 to 18 month olds presenting with FSFS?

Answer
Not routinely. In fully vaccinated children with FSFS, the risk of bacterial meningitis without other symptoms or focality is extremely low.

Reference
1. Subcommittee on Febrile Seizures; American Academy of Pediatrics. Neurodiagnostic evaluation of the child with a simple febrile seizure. *Pediatrics.* 2011;127(2):389–394.

ORAL ONDANSETRON FOR GASTROENTERITIS

CHAPTER 22

Thomas F. Heyne ■ Lauren Allister

Oral Ondansetron for Gastroenteritis in a Pediatric Emergency Department
Freedman SB, Adler M, Seshadri R, et al. *N Engl J Med.* 2006;354(16):1698–1705

BACKGROUND
Acute gastroenteritis is estimated to account for >1.5 million outpatient visits and 200,000 hospitalizations in the US annually.[1] Oral rehydration therapy (ORT) for mild-to-moderate dehydration has been recommended both by the Centers for Disease Control and Prevention and the American Academy of Pediatrics, but physicians are sometimes hesitant to initiate oral fluids and medications in an actively vomiting patient.[1,2] Prior to this study, there were limited data on the benefit of adding the antiemetic ondansetron as an adjunct to ORT in the acute setting.

OBJECTIVES
To determine if administration of a single oral disintegrating tablet (ODT) of ondansetron decreases vomiting or improves clinical outcomes in children with gastroenteritis receiving ORT for mild-to-moderate dehydration.

METHODS
Double-blind, randomized controlled trial in an academic pediatric emergency department (ED) from 2004 to 2005.

Patients
215 children ages 6 months to 10 years presenting with ≥1 episode of nonbloody, nonbilious emesis within the preceding 4 hours, ≥1 episode of diarrhea, and mild-to-moderate dehydration. Select exclusion criteria: severe dehydration, weight <8 kg, or prior abdominal surgery.

Intervention
Patients were randomized to receive a weight-based dose of ondansetron ODT or placebo, followed by a second dose if the patient vomited within 15 minutes of initial dose. After 15 minutes, a 1-hour period of intense ORT was completed (<30 cc of electrolyte solution administered by caregivers every 5 minutes) until disposition was determined, after which the physician resumed usual care. The child's family was telephoned at 3 and 7 days post intervention.

Outcomes
Primary outcome was vomiting during ORT. Secondary outcomes included number of vomiting episodes, need for IV hydration, and hospitalization.

KEY RESULTS

- Vomiting during ORT occurred significantly less often in the ondansetron group as compared to placebo (14% vs. 35%; RR = 0.40, 95% CI 0.26–0.61).
- Children who received ondansetron had fewer episodes of vomiting (RR = 0.30, 95% CI 0.18–0.50), had greater oral intake (239 mL vs. 196 mL, p = 0.001), and were less likely to require IV hydration (RR 0.46, 95% CI 0.26–0.79).
- Mean length of ED stay was 12% shorter in the ondansetron group (p = 0.02), although there was no significant difference in hospitalization rates or return visits.
- Children receiving ondansetron had more episodes of diarrhea (1.4 vs. 0.5, p < 0.01), but no other adverse events.

STUDY CONCLUSIONS

A single dose of ondansetron ODT in children with gastroenteritis and mild-to-moderate dehydration decreased vomiting and facilitated successful ORT.

COMMENTARY

This study affirms that vomiting is not a contraindication to ORT, demonstrating that a single dose of ODT ondansetron improves the success of oral rehydration, decreasing vomiting, and need for IV hydration by over 50%. Study limitations included the use of an unvalidated dehydration score and a limited period of ED observation. In 2011, a Cochrane review of 7 trials confirmed these findings and also showed a reduction in hospital admissions, establishing this practice as an accepted standard of care.[3]

Question

Does ondansetron improve ORT in patients with mild-to-moderate dehydration caused by gastroenteritis?

Answer

Yes. Ondansetron decreases vomiting during oral rehydration and need for IV hydration.

ACKNOWLEDGMENT

We would like to thank Dr. Kathryn Hawk for her contributions to this chapter.

References

1. King CK, Glass R, Bresee JS, et al.; Centers for Disease Control and Prevention. Managing acute gastroenteritis among children: Oral rehydration, maintenance, and nutritional therapy. *MMWR Recomm Rep.* 2003;52(RR-16):1–16.
2. Ozuah PO, Avner JR, Stein RE. Oral rehydration, emergency physicians, and practice parameters: A national survey. *Pediatrics.* 2002;109(2):259–261.
3. Fedorowicz Z, Jagannath VA, Carter B. Antiemetics for reducing vomiting related to acute gastroenteritis in children and adolescents. *Cochrane Database Syst Rev.* 2011;(9):CD005506.

CHAPTER 23

ORAL VERSUS INTRAVENOUS
REHYDRATION

Emily M. Herzberg ■ Lauren Allister

Oral Versus Intravenous Rehydration of Moderately Dehydrated Children: A
Randomized, Controlled Trial

Spandorfer PR, Alessandrini EA, Joffe MD, et al. *Pediatrics*. 2005;115(2):
295–301

BACKGROUND
Acute gastroenteritis is a major cause of morbidity in the US, estimated to account for
>1.5 million outpatient visits and 200,000 hospitalizations.[1] Oral rehydration therapy
(ORT) had previously been recommended by the American Academy of Pediatrics
(AAP) and World Health Organization (WHO) as first-line therapy for children with
mild-to-moderate dehydration. However, many pediatric emergency department (ED)
providers were using IV rehydration due to perceived ease, the presence of vomiting,
resources involved in administering ORT, and presumed parental expectations.[2] This
study aimed to evaluate the effectiveness of ORT as compared to IV rehydration in pediatric patients presenting to the ED with gastroenteritis and moderate dehydration.

OBJECTIVES
To determine whether ORT is effective in treatment of moderate dehydration as compared to IV hydration.

METHODS
Single-blind, randomized controlled noninferiority study conducted in a single US
pediatric ED from 2001 to 2003.

Patients
73 patients ages 8 weeks to 3 years with moderate dehydration (5% to 10% dehydration as
determined by a 10-point scale) and diagnosis of probable viral gastroenteritis (≥3 loose
or watery stools in the previous 24 hours). Select exclusion criteria: hypotension, >5 days
of illness, recent ED treatment, malnutrition, failure to thrive, impaired oromotor skills.

Intervention
Electrolyte solution ORT in fixed aliquots over 4 hours totaling 50 mL/kg or 75 mL/kg
depending on baseline degree of dehydration. IV hydration group received two 20 mL/kg
normal saline IV boluses within the first hour, and were then encouraged to drink oral fluids
for the remaining 3 hours.

Outcomes
Primary outcome was success of treatment at 4 hours, defined as resolution of moderate
dehydration, weight gain, urine production, and absence of severe emesis during the last

hour of the trial. Secondary outcomes were time to initiation of therapy, improvement in dehydration score after 2 hours, hospitalization rate, parental preference, and ED return visits within 72 hours.

KEY RESULTS

- ORT demonstrated noninferiority with 55.6% of ORT and 56.8% of IV hydration patients successfully rehydrated at 4 hours (difference: −1.2%, 95% CI −24–21.6).
- Time to initiate therapy was significantly shorter in the ORT group as compared to the IV hydration group (19.9 minutes vs. 41.2 minutes, 95% CI 10.3–32.1).

STUDY CONCLUSIONS

ORT was as effective as IV fluid in rehydration of moderately dehydrated young children secondary to gastroenteritis and was faster to initiate.

COMMENTARY

This study demonstrates that ORT is easily implemented in the ED setting and produces equivalent outcomes to IV rehydration. ORT confers important clinical benefits including faster time to initiation and avoidance of painful procedures. Additionally, parents can be educated to employ this skill effectively at home. This study showed a trend toward fewer hospitalizations among ORT patients and improved parental satisfaction, although these findings did not reach statistical significance. This study was stopped early due to a decline in enrollment as ORT became the gold standard.

Question

Is oral rehydration as effective as IV rehydration in children with moderate dehydration secondary to gastroenteritis in the pediatric ED?

Answer

Yes, oral rehydration is as effective as IV fluids, easy to administer and teach to parents, and reduces painful procedures in children.

References

1. King CK, Glass R, Bresee JS, et al.; Centers for Disease Control and Prevention. Managing acute gastroenteritis among children: Oral rehydration, maintenance, and nutritional therapy. *MMWR Recomm Rep.* 2003;52(RR-16):1–16.
2. Ozuah PO, Avner JR, Stein RE. Oral rehydration, emergency physicians, and practice parameters: A national survey. *Pediatrics.* 2002;109(2):259–261.

CHAPTER 24

ORAL DEXAMETHASONE FOR MILD CROUP

Emily M. Herzberg ■ Lauren Allister

A Randomized Trial of a Single Dose of Oral Dexamethasone for Mild Croup
Bjornson CL, Klassen TP, Williamson J, et al. *N Engl J Med.* 2004;351(13):1306–1313

BACKGROUND

Croup (acute laryngotracheobronchitis) is a common presenting complaint in the emergency department (ED). 60% of these children have mild symptoms (barking cough and no stridor at rest) and can be discharged without treatment given an expected uncomplicated course. Previous studies evaluating oral corticosteroid use focused on children with moderate-to-severe symptoms of croup. This study aimed to assess the benefits of corticosteroids in mild disease.

OBJECTIVES

To evaluate the benefits of a single dose of oral dexamethasone in children with mild croup.

METHODS

Double-blind, randomized, placebo-controlled trial in 4 pediatric EDs in Canada from 2001 to 2003.

Patients

720 children ages 1 to 5 years with mild croup (onset of barking cough within previous 72 hours and score <2 on the Westley croup scale).[1] Select exclusion criteria: alternative cause of stridor, chronic lung disease, systemic disease, immune dysfunction, or recent treatment with corticosteroids.

Intervention

Administration of a single dose of oral dexamethasone (0.6 mg/kg, maximum dose of 20 mg) vs. similarly flavored placebo. Parental surveys were administered.

Outcomes

Primary outcome was return to any medical provider within 7 days. Secondary outcomes included time to symptom resolution, costs, hours of child's lost sleep, and parental stress.

KEY RESULTS

- Return to healthcare provider within 7 days was higher in the placebo vs. dexamethasone group (15.3% vs. 7.3%, 95% CI 3.3–12.5). Number needed to treat (NNT) to prevent 1 return visit was 13 (95% CI 8–31).

- Dexamethasone group had quicker symptom resolution ($p = 0.003$), less sleep loss ($p < 0.001$), $21 average savings per case ($p = 0.01$), and less parental stress on day 1 post treatment ($p < 0.001$). There was no difference in reported stress on days 2 and 3.
- Placebo group had greater severity of croup in the first 24 hours as compared to the dexamethasone group (95% CI 1.5–6.8), although this difference largely disappeared by 72 hours.

STUDY CONCLUSIONS

A single dose of oral dexamethasone reduced return visits and croup symptoms within 24 hours of treatment, in addition to decreasing cost and parental stress.

COMMENTARY

The majority of children with croup have mild symptoms, and this study was one of the first to demonstrate the clinical, social, and economic benefits of dexamethasone administration in this population which helped shape current clinical practice. Limitations included lack of investigation into common side effects of dexamethasone and insufficient power to examine for any serious adverse effects. Notably, this study allowed a maximum dose of 20 mg of dexamethasone, while current practice recommends no more than 10 mg for a single dose. These data were corroborated by the 2012 Cochrane review that demonstrated corticosteroid treatment in croup results in decreased return visits, readmissions, and overall time spent in the hospital.[2]

Question

Does a single oral dose of dexamethasone (0.6 mg/kg) in mild croup improve symptom recovery and decrease return medical visits?

Answer

Yes, children with mild croup treated with a single dose of dexamethasone are more likely to have improved symptoms within 24 hours and less likely to return to a healthcare provider within 7 days.

ACKNOWLEDGMENT

We would like to thank Dr. Radhika Sundararajan for her contributions to this chapter.

References

1. Westley CR, Cotton EK, Brooks JG. Nebulized racemic epinephrine by IPPB for the treatment of croup: A double-blind study. *Am J Dis Child.* 1978;132(5):484–487.
2. Russell KF, Liang Y, O'Gorman K, et al. Glucocorticoids for croup. *Cochrane Database Syst Rev.* 2011; (1):CD001955.

LIKELIHOOD OF OCCULT PNEUMONIA IN FEBRILE CHILDREN

CHAPTER 25

Emily M. Herzberg ■ Lauren Allister

Occult Pneumonias: Empiric Chest Radiographs in Febrile Children With Leukocytosis
Bachur R, Perry H, Harper MB. *Ann Emerg Med.* 1999;33(2):166–173

BACKGROUND
The evaluation of febrile children is diagnostically challenging. In febrile children with leukocytosis and respiratory symptoms, chest radiographs (CXRs) are often performed to evaluate for underlying pneumonia. However, performance of CXR in febrile children without respiratory symptoms was not standard practice. This study was the first to examine the utility of CXR in febrile children with no clinically identifiable source.

OBJECTIVES
To evaluate the incidence of radiographic pneumonia in children with fever and leukocytosis without a source of infection on examination.

METHODS
Prospective cohort study at a single US center from 1994 to 1995.

Patients
278 patients ages <5 years with leukocytosis (white blood cell [WBC] count >20,000/mm^3) and temperature >39.0°C. Select exclusion criteria: immunodeficiency, chronic lung disease, identified source of major bacterial infection (otitis media not included).

Intervention
Pneumonia diagnosed by CXR in children without respiratory signs (tachypnea, increased work of breathing, oxygen desaturation) in comparison to children who underwent CXR due to clinical concern for pneumonia.

Outcomes
Primary outcome was diagnosis of occult pneumonia.

KEY RESULTS
- Occult pneumonia was identified in 26% (95% CI 19–34) and 31% (95% CI 20–44) of children with WBC counts of >20,000/mm^3 and >25,000/mm^3, respectively. In comparison, 41% (95% CI 30–52) of symptomatic children were diagnosed with pneumonia.

- Assuming all children without CXR did not have pneumonia, minimum estimates of occult pneumonia were 19% (95% CI 14–25) and 26% (95% CI 16–39) in patients with WBC counts >20,000/mm^3 and >25,000/mm^3, respectively.
- No individual sign or constellation of clinical findings was a sensitive predictor of pneumonia.

STUDY CONCLUSIONS

Empiric CXRs should be considered routinely in the evaluation of highly febrile children with leukocytosis and no identifiable source of infection; approximately 20% of these patients had an occult pneumonia.

COMMENTARY

While the overall incidence of pneumococcal pneumonia may be lower in pediatric patients in the post-conjugate vaccine era,[1] multiple subsequent pediatric emergency department studies have confirmed the importance of this study's findings.[2,3] Limitations included reliance on the WBC alone to inform decision making without providing the indication for obtaining the CBC as well as this not being standard of practice. The incidence of occult pneumonia in this study population supports the routine use of CXR for highly febrile patients with leukocytosis, even in the absence of respiratory symptoms.

Question

Should chest radiography be routinely performed in the evaluation of children with high fever and leukocytosis but no identified source of infection?

Answer

Yes, imaging should be considered in the evaluation of febrile children with WBC counts >20,000/mm^3, even without respiratory symptoms, as a significant number will have occult pneumonia.

References

1. Loo JD, Conklin L, Fleming-Dutra KE, et al. Systematic review of the effect of pneumococcal conjugate vaccine dosing schedules on prevention of pneumonia. *Pediatr Infect Dis J.* 2014;33 (Suppl 2):S140–S151.
2. Mintegi S, Benito J, Pijoan JI, et al. Occult pneumonia in infants with high fever without source: A prospective multicenter study. *Pediatr Emerg Care.* 2010;26(7):470–474.
3. Rutman MS, Bachur R, Harper MB. Radiographic pneumonia in young, highly febrile children with leukocytosis before and after universal conjugate pneumococcal vaccination. *Pediatr Emerg Care.* 2009;25(1): 1–7.

IPRATROPIUM IN ACUTE ASTHMA MANAGEMENT

CHAPTER 26

Emily M. Herzberg ■ Lauren Allister

Ipratropium Bromide Added to Asthma Treatment in the Pediatric Emergency Department

Zorc JJ, Pusic MV, Ogborn CJ, et al. *Pediatrics.* 1999;103(4):748–752

BACKGROUND

Asthma affects approximately 9.3% of children in the US and accounts for 1.8 million pediatric emergency department (ED) visits annually.[1] Prior to this study, standard asthma therapy in the ED included high-dose inhaled beta-agonists and systemic corticosteroids. Ipratropium had been well studied as an adjunctive agent in adults with proven improvement in bronchodilation and forced expiratory volume in 1 second (FEV1). However, the efficacy of ipratropium in the treatment of pediatric asthma was not well known.

OBJECTIVES

To measure the effect of the addition of ipratropium to standard asthma therapy (3 nebulized albuterol treatments and oral corticosteroids) in the pediatric ED.

METHODS

Double-blind, randomized placebo-controlled trial in a single US pediatric ED from 1997 to 1998.

Patients

365 children ages >12 months (427 visits) presenting to the ED with wheezing and treated according to a pre-existing clinical pathway for asthma. Select exclusion criteria: respiratory failure, requirement of therapy beyond standard pathway, recent oral corticosteroid or ipratropium use, cystic fibrosis.

Intervention

Ipratropium 250 μg/dose vs. equivalent volume of normal saline was administered with each of the first 3 nebulized albuterol treatments (2.5 mg if <30 kg or 5 mg if >30 kg, each 20 minutes apart). Participants additionally received 2 mg/kg (80 mg maximum) of oral prednisone or prednisolone within the first hour of therapy. After the first hour, additional therapy was at physicians' discretion. Further ipratropium was avoided unless patients were clinically worsening or admitted. Asthma severity score (based on accessory muscle use, wheeze, and dyspnea) was assessed on an ongoing basis.

Outcomes

Primary outcomes were disposition (home, ward admission, or intensive care unit admission), and, for discharged patients, number of nebulizer treatments received and time-to-discharge. Secondary outcomes included ED return visits <72 hours and hospital charges incurred by discharged patients.

KEY RESULTS

- Mean time-to-discharge was 28 minutes shorter in the patients with mild-to-moderate severity scores treated with ipratropium as compared to the control group ($p = 0.001$).
- Fewer albuterol nebulizer treatments were required in the ipratropium group as compared to the control group (median of 3 vs. 4 treatments, $p < 0.01$).

STUDY CONCLUSIONS

The addition of ipratropium to albuterol and corticosteroids in the treatment of asthma in the pediatric ED was associated with reduction in time-to-discharge and number of nebulizer treatments required.

COMMENTARY

This study was the first to examine the use of ipratropium and its effects on pediatric asthma outcomes in the ED. These results are the basis for the use of "stacked" or combined nebulizer treatments (3 treatments of ipratropium and albuterol administered every 20 minutes), now an accepted standard for acute asthma care. In the ipratropium group, there was also a trend toward fewer hospital admissions, although this was not statistically significant. Of note, while ipratropium is routinely used in initial ED therapy, it is not recommended for ongoing administration in pediatric patients. Additionally, the currently recommended maximum dose of corticosteroids is now 60 mg rather than the 80 mg used in this study.

Question

Does the addition of ipratropium improve standard asthma therapy among pediatric patients in the ED?

Answer

Yes, the addition of ipratropium to standard acute asthma therapy, as "stacked" nebulizers combined with albuterol, shortens time-to-discharge from the ED and reduces the total number of albuterol doses needed.

Reference

1. Bloom B, Jones LI, Freeman G. Summary health statistics for U.S. children: National Health Interview Survey, 2012. *Vital Health Stat 10.* 2013;(258):1–81.

CHAPTER 27

EVALUATION OF THE FEBRILE INFANT

Emily M. Herzberg ■ Lauren Allister

Identification of Infants Unlikely to Have Serious Bacterial Infection Although Hospitalized for Suspected Sepsis

Dagan R, Powell KR, Hall CB, et al. *J Pediatr.* 1985;107(6):855–860 **(Rochester group)**

Outpatient Treatment of Febrile Infants 28 to 89 Days of Age With Intramuscular Administration of Ceftriaxone

Baskin MN, O'Rourke EJ, Fleisher GR. *J Pediatr.* 1992;120(1):22–27 **(Boston group)**

Outpatient Management Without Antibiotics of Fever in Selected Infants

Baker MD, Bell LM, Avner JR. *N Engl J Med.* 1993;329(20):1437–1441 **(Philadelphia group)**

BACKGROUND

The evaluation and management of the febrile infant <3 months of age has been debated for decades. The prevalence of serious bacterial infection (SBI) in infants 0 to 3 months with fever is approximately 8%, with the highest prevalence (25%) in infants <2 weeks.[1] Determining which febrile infants have an underlying SBI cannot be ascertained solely based on clinical appearance, often necessitating invasive diagnostic testing. Prior to these studies, common practice had been to hospitalize infants <3 months of age for evaluation, antibiotic administration, and observation, which was costly, time consuming, and resource heavy. These landmark investigations were the first to suggest possible pathways for risk stratification of young febrile infants.

	Rochester group	Boston group	Philadelphia group
Objectives	To determine whether results of physical examination, WBC/band count, and UA could predict and stratify risk for SBI.	To determine outcomes of outpatient management of febrile infants at low risk of occult bacteremia with administration of IM CTX.	To evaluate the efficacy and costs of management of febrile infants without empiric antibiotics or routine hospitalization.
Methods	Single center, prospective, cohort study in an ED from 1982 to 1984.	Single center, prospective, consecutive cohort study in a pediatric ED from 1987 to 1990.	Single center, prospective, randomized trial in a pediatric ED from 1987 to 1992.

	Rochester group	Boston group	Philadelphia group
Patients	233 previously healthy infants age <89 d hospitalized for sepsis evaluation, stratified to low- and high-risk groups. Infants classified as low risk: • No obvious source of infection • Peripheral WBC count 5,000–15,000/mm^3 • <1,500 bands/mm^3 • UA <10 WBCs/hpf • No recent antibiotic therapy CXR and CSF results were not used for risk stratification.	503 infants ages 28–89 d with: • Well appearance • Rectal temperature ≥38°C • No obvious source of infection • Peripheral WBC count <20,000 cells/µL • Urinalysis with <10 WBCs/hpf or dipstick negative for leukocyte esterase • CSF WBC count <10 cells/µL • No infiltrate on CXR if obtained • No other admission indication • No antibiotics in the prior 48 h	747 infants ages 29–56 d, with rectal temperatures ≥38.2°C, stratified to low- or high-risk, and treated with inpatient or outpatient observation or empiric antibiotics. Infants deemed low-risk (148 inpatient, 139 outpatient): • No obvious source of infection • Peripheral WBC <15,000/mm^3 • Urinalysis with <10 WBCs/hpf • CSF <8 WBCs/mm^3 • No infiltrate on CXR
Intervention	Performance of CBC/differential, UA, LP; blood, urine, and CSF cultures. Viral/stool swabs and CXR obtained dependent on season and symptoms. All were hospitalized and 200 received parenteral antibiotics.	Performance of CBC/differential, UA, LP; blood, urine, CSF, stool cultures. CXR at physicians' discretion. 50 mg/kg CTX IM then administered with return at 24 h for second dose. Follow-up by phone at 48 h and 7 d.	Performance of CBC/differential, UA, LP; blood, urine, CSF cultures; CXR. Stool culture/WBCs if diarrhea. Infants at high-risk were admitted and received antibiotics. Low-risk infants were randomized to outpatient management without antibiotics or inpatient observation without antibiotics. Reevaluation occurred at 24 and 48 h.
Outcomes	Incidence of SBI among low-risk compared to high-risk infants, and clinical and laboratory findings predictive of SBI.	Incidence of SBI among infants discharged home after IM CTX, and factors predictive of SBI.	Incidence of SBI among low-risk compared to high-risk infants and cost of treatment.

	Rochester group	Boston group	Philadelphia group
Key Results	• 0.7% (1/144) of infants in the low-risk group had SBI compared with 25% (22/89) of infants in the high-risk group (*p* <0.0001). • No low-risk infants had bacteremia, compared with 10% of high-risk infants (*p* <0.0001). • NPV of screening criteria was 99.3% for SBI and 100% for sepsis. • 60% of infants with SBI had temperatures >39°C, compared to 39% of the other group (*p* = 0.04).	• 5.4% (27/503) febrile infants had SBI. • Temperature (*p* <0.01) and absolute and percentage of band forms (*p* <0.001) were higher in febrile infants with SBI, compared to those without SBI. • 13/25 infants with SBI would have been identified as high risk by Rochester criteria (sensitivity = 0.52).	• 99.7% (286/287) of infants assigned to observation without anti-biotics did not have an SBI. • Sensitivity of SBI screen-ing was 98% (95% CI 92–100) and NPV was 99.7% (95% CI 98–100). • Only 2 infants receiving outpatient treatment required subsequent hospitalization for other indications; neither had SBI. • Outpatient observation saved $2,500/patient compared to inpatient observation.
Study Conclusions	Laboratory criteria were successfully used to identify infants <89 d undergoing sepsis evaluations without clinical evidence of infection who were at low risk for SBI and could be carefully observed inpatient without antibiotics.	Outpatient manage-ment with 48 h of IM CTX after a full sepsis evaluation (including at minimum CBC, UA, LP, blood/urine/ CSF cultures) in infants 29–89 d with a strict follow-up protocol was a safe alternative to hospital admission.	Infants 29–56 d at low risk for SBI based on sepsis evaluation (including CBC, UA, LP, and blood/urine/ CSF cultures), can be safely and effectively managed at home without antibiotics.

Abbreviations: CBC, complete blood count; CSF, cerebrospinal fluid; CTX, ceftriaxone; CXR, chest x-ray; d, days; h, hours; hpf, high power field; IM, intramuscular; LP, lumbar puncture; SBI, serious bacterial infection; UA, urinalysis; WBC, white blood cell count.

COMMENTARY

The Rochester, Boston, and Philadelphia studies have served as the foundation for guidance in the management of febrile infants <3 months old and underscore the importance of WBC count with differential, UA, CSF cell counts, and overall clini-cal appearance as major predictors of the likelihood of SBI. The Rochester group was the first to evaluate management of young febrile infants, but given that all patients were admitted with the majority receiving antibiotics, it was challenging to extrapolate the findings to outpatient management. The Boston group subsequently demonstrated the success of outpatient management in low-risk febrile infants. However, all patients received antibiotics, introducing the potential for medica-tion side effects, high cost, antibiotic resistance, and the need to complete a lumbar puncture prior to treatment even in well-appearing infants. Finally, the Philadelphia group provided data to support outpatient management without antibiotics, still requiring substantial invasive testing prior to risk stratification. For febrile infants <29 days, the accepted standard of care remains a full sepsis evaluation (including

LP), inpatient observation, and antibiotics. Infants 1 to 3 months can be safely managed as outpatients with consideration of antibiotics after risk stratification based on blood and urine studies. The recommendation for performance of an LP in this age group varies, most notably in the 2- to 3-month age group, allowing for provider and institutional variability. In the post-conjugate vaccine era and with development of newer inflammatory markers (e.g., procalcitonin), risk stratification and management strategies for young febrile infants will continue to evolve.

Question

Can febrile infants <3 months be successfully identified as low risk for SBI and subsequently managed as outpatients (with or without antibiotics)?

Answer

Yes, the Boston, Philadelphia, or Rochester criteria can be used. Low-risk infants 1 to 3 months can be successfully managed as outpatients with close follow-up. These infants require some invasive testing (complete blood count with differential, urinalysis, urine and blood cultures) but do not always require lumbar puncture or further testing depending on age, appearance, and vaccination status.

ACKNOWLEDGMENT

We would like to thank Dr. Kito Lord for his contributions to this chapter.

Reference

1. Hui C, Neto G, Tsertsvadze A, et al. Diagnosis and management of febrile infants (0-3 months). *Evid Rep Technol Assess (Full Rep).* 2012;205:1–297.

SECTION 5

ENDOCRINOLOGY

5

28. Maintenance of Glycemic Control in Type 2 Diabetes
29. Impact of Body Mass Index on Pubertal Development
30. Cerebral Edema in Diabetic Ketoacidosis
31. Intensive Insulin Treatment for Type 1 Diabetes
32. Prevention of Intellectual Impairment With Neonatal
   Hypothyroidism Screening

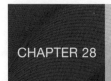

MAINTENANCE OF GLYCEMIC CONTROL IN TYPE 2 DIABETES

CHAPTER 28

Mary Perry Alexander ■ Takara Stanley

A Clinical Trial to Maintain Glycemic Control in Youth With Type 2 Diabetes

TODAY (Type 2 Diabetes in Adolescents and Youth) Study Group

Zeitler P, Hirst K, Pyle L, et al. *N Engl J Med.* 2012;366(24):2247–2256

BACKGROUND

In youth, along with a dramatic rise in obesity, the prevalence of type 2 diabetes mellitus (T2DM) has increased since the 1990s. Because organ-damaging vascular disease from hyperglycemia accrues over time, it is particularly important to achieve glycemic control in children, but there was previously little evidence to guide this.

OBJECTIVES

To evaluate whether combination therapy with metformin and rosiglitazone would provide improved glycemic control in youth with recent-onset T2DM as compared to metformin alone, or metformin + lifestyle modification.

METHODS

Randomized clinical trial conducted at 15 US centers from 2004 to 2011.

Patients

699 patients ages 10 to 17 years with T2DM for <2 years, negative diabetes-related autoantibodies, and body mass index (BMI) ≥85th percentile. Select exclusion criteria: renal or hepatic impairment, steroid use, pregnancy.

Intervention

Comparison of 1,000 mg metformin twice daily with metformin + 4 mg rosiglitazone twice daily or metformin + intensive lifestyle intervention (weekly in-person contact with lifestyle coach for 6 months, 200 to 300 minutes of physical activity per week, 1,200 to 1,500 kcal/d diet). Mean follow-up was 3.8 years. Medication intervention was double blinded.

Outcomes

Primary outcome was time to treatment failure (hemoglobin A1c [HbA1c] ≥8% over 6 months, or inability to wean from insulin, if started for metabolic decompensation). Secondary outcomes included BMI, lipid levels, blood pressure, insulin sensitivity, and albumin-to-creatinine ratio.

KEY RESULTS
- 45.6% of all participants had treatment failure, with a median time to failure of 11.5 months.

- Metformin + rosiglitazone had the lowest failure rate (38.6%, 95% CI 32.4–44.9) compared to metformin alone (51.7%, 95% CI 45.3–58.2) and metformin + lifestyle (46.6%, 95% CI 40.2–53.0). In direct comparison, metformin alone and metformin + lifestyle were indistinguishable ($p = 0.17$).
- Patients receiving metformin + rosiglitazone had the greatest increase in BMI; metformin + lifestyle group had the least ($p < 0.001$).
- There were 4 episodes of severe hypoglycemia overall. Although 19.2% of patients reported serious adverse events, 87% of these were considered unrelated to study treatment.

STUDY CONCLUSIONS

Metformin monotherapy provided durable glycemic control in <50% of children and adolescents with new-onset T2DM. While addition of rosiglitazone decreased failure rates, there was no incremental improvement provided by intensive lifestyle intervention.

COMMENTARY

The TODAY study, suggesting that T2DM progressed to insulin dependence rapidly in the majority of youth, was disheartening to providers, as adolescents had significantly increased failure rates with metformin monotherapy compared to the reported <20% per year in adults.[1] Subsequent studies from this cohort suggest that rapid progression of T2DM in youth may result from accelerated deterioration of beta-cell function; strategies to slow the loss are under investigation. The most promising arm of the study, metformin combined with rosiglitazone, is not recommended due to the "black box" warning on rosiglitazone for increased risk of congestive heart failure. The lack of additional efficacy from adding an intensive lifestyle intervention to metformin was also discouraging, particularly given that the intervention was evidence based and quite intensive. Presently, metformin with lifestyle modifications remains the recommended initial therapy for adolescents with T2DM unless HbA1c ≥9%.

Question
What is the most effective therapy for youth with newly diagnosed type 2 diabetes?

Answer
There is not an effective therapy to delay need for insulin in the majority of the population. Metformin with an intensive lifestyle intervention is the current recommended initial therapy, but achieves glycemic control in only ~50% of youth.

Reference
1. Brown JB, Conner C, Nichols GA. Secondary failure of metformin monotherapy in clinical practice. *Diabetes Care.* 2010;33(3):501–506.

IMPACT OF BODY MASS INDEX ON PUBERTAL DEVELOPMENT

Mary Perry Alexander ■ Takara Stanley

Thelarche, Pubarche, and Menarche Attainment in Children With Normal and Elevated Body Mass Index

Rosenfield RL, Lipton RB, Drum ML. *Pediatrics*. 2009;123(1):84–88

BACKGROUND

The normal timing of puberty among US children has been debated. Prior studies noted differences in puberty onset based on ethnicity and obesity, but these studies had methodologic limitations and were not sufficiently conclusive to modify definitions of early puberty (before age 8 in girls or age 9 in boys). This study was designed to measure timing of key pubertal milestones and examine the association with elevated body mass index (BMI).

OBJECTIVES

To determine the age of key pubertal milestones in US girls with normal BMI versus those with BMI ≥85th percentile, and assess the age of pubarche in US boys.

METHODS

Retrospective analysis of National Health and Nutrition Examination Survey (NHANES) III data (a large study that randomly surveyed the US population on health-related issues) from 1988 to 1994.

Patients

1,914 girls were assessed for age at thelarche (breast stage 2); 1,888 girls and 1,869 boys were assessed for age at pubarche (pubic hair stage 3); and 2,065 girls were assessed for age at menarche (onset of menses). Select exclusion criterion: severe mental or physical impairment.

Intervention

Analysis of data on race/ethnicity and pubertal assessments from examination with inspection for pubertal signs, questionnaire, and NHANES III.

Outcomes

Primary outcomes were age at onset of thelarche, pubarche, and menarche.

KEY RESULTS

- Thelarche was observed in only 3.2% of 8-year-old girls with normal BMI. Of these, 19.2% of Mexican-American (MA) girls and 12.1% of non-Hispanic black (NHB) girls attained breast development by age 8, as compared to 1.3% of non-Hispanic white (NHW) girls.

- Girls with BMI ≥85% had a higher prevalence of thelarche from ages 8 to 9.6 years (OR 3.86, 95% CI 1.16–12.9) than girls with BMI <85% (OR 2.02, 95% CI 1.00–4.08), and their median age of menarche was 5.4 months earlier.
- Pubarche occurred in <3% of girls under age 8 with normal BMI, regardless of ethnicity.
- BMI ≥85% was associated with increased rates of pubarche between ages 8 (OR 4.5, 95% CI 1.52–13.3) and 10.2 (OR 1.87, 95% CI 1.02–3.43) in girls, but there was no association between adiposity and pubarche in boys.

STUDY CONCLUSIONS

Increased BMI was associated with earlier average age of pubertal milestones in girls, but not with pubarche in boys. Thelarche occurred earlier on average in NHB and MA girls compared to NHW girls, such that thelarche before age 8 appeared to be typical in these groups.

COMMENTARY

This study helped to redefine classification of pubertal development in girls. Previously, any pubertal changes before age 8 were considered premature, often prompting investigation such as bone age radiography and laboratory assessments. Based on this study and others, clinicians now use BMI (a proxy for adiposity) and ethnicity in defining norms. Limitations include the exclusion of other ethnic groups, as well as the ascertainment of breast development by inspection rather than palpation, which may cause adipomastia to be misidentified as thelarche. Importantly, this study showed that thelarche before age 8 may be normal in NHB or MA girls, and in overweight girls of any ethnicity. Although tracking of pubertal development in these children is still advised, if changes progress as expected further investigation may not be indicated. Why BMI is associated with earlier pubertal development in girls but not boys remains unclear.

Question

Does BMI or race/ethnicity impact the timing of pubertal changes?

Answer

Yes. BMI ≥ 85%, as well as NHB or MA ethnic background are associated with earlier thelarche in girls.

CHAPTER 30

CEREBRAL EDEMA IN DIABETIC KETOACIDOSIS

Mary Perry Alexander ■ Takara Stanley

Risk Factors for Cerebral Edema in Children With Diabetic Ketoacidosis

Glaser NG, Barnett IM, McCaslin I, et al. *N Engl J Med.* 2001;344(4):264–269

BACKGROUND

Cerebral edema is a dreaded complication of diabetic ketoacidosis (DKA) and the most common cause of DKA-related mortality. Prior to this study, only a few small clinical studies had elucidated risk factors for cerebral edema in children presenting with DKA: younger age, new diabetes diagnosis, and faster fluid resuscitation rates. The potential effect of other factors, particularly therapeutic interventions, had yet to be assessed in large cohorts.

OBJECTIVES

To identify the risk factors associated with development of cerebral edema among children presenting with DKA.

METHODS

Retrospective, case-controlled study at 10 US pediatric centers from 1982 to 1997.

Patients

416 patients ≤18 years old with DKA (serum glucose >300 mg/dL, venous pH <7.25 or serum bicarbonate <15 mmol/L, and ketonuria). This included 61 cases with cerebral edema, 174 matched controls without cerebral edema, and 181 random controls without cerebral edema.

Intervention

Comparison of demographic characteristics, initial biochemical values, treatment regimen, and changes in laboratory values during treatment between the groups.

Outcomes

Clinical characteristics and treatment strategies were compared between children who did and did not develop cerebral edema.

KEY RESULTS

- Compared to random controls, patients who developed cerebral edema were more likely to be young (8.9 years vs. 11.3 years, $p < 0.001$), white (73% vs. 53%, $p = 0.009$), and recently diagnosed with diabetes (66% vs. 39%, $p < 0.001$).
- Patients with cerebral edema had lower initial partial pressures of arterial carbon dioxide ($PaCO_2$) (RR 2.7 for each 7.8 mm Hg decrease, 95% CI 1.4–5.1) and

higher serum urea nitrogen concentrations (RR 1.8 for each 9 mg/dL increase, 95% CI 1.2–2.7) as compared to matched controls.
- The only therapeutic intervention associated with increased risk of cerebral edema compared to matched controls was bicarbonate administration (RR 4.2, 95% CI 1.5–12.1).
- Patients with cerebral edema had smaller increases in serum sodium concentrations during therapy (RR 0.6 per increase of 5.8 mmol/L/h, 95% CI 0.4–0.9) as compared to matched controls.

STUDY CONCLUSIONS

Low arterial $PaCO_2$, high serum urea nitrogen, lack of serum sodium increase during treatment, and administration of bicarbonate were associated with increased risk for development of cerebral edema in patients with DKA.

COMMENTARY

This study sought to rigorously examine the risk factors associated with cerebral edema by controlling for covariates in a way that prior studies had not. Unlike other studies, this one did not find the expected associations between rates of fluid, insulin, or sodium administration and cerebral edema. Rather than bolstering the previously held idea that cerebral edema was iatrogenic and due to osmotically mediated swelling, the identified risk factors supported a model of brain ischemia secondary to hypocapneic vasoconstriction and extreme dehydration. Based on this study, bicarbonate therapy should be employed only in the setting of severe acidosis (pH < 6.9) or impending cardiovascular collapse. All children presenting in DKA, particularly those with risk factors of low $PaCO_2$, high serum urea nitrogen concentrations, and persistently low serum sodium concentrations during therapy, should be monitored closely for evidence of neurologic impairment and treated immediately with hyperosmolar therapy if concerns arise. Comprehensive DKA guidelines were published in 2014.[1]

Question

Which therapies should be avoided in children with DKA due to increased risk of development of cerebral edema?

Answer

In this study, bicarbonate therapy was the only treatment associated with development of cerebral edema, and is only recommended in cases of severe acidosis (pH < 6.9) or impending cardiovascular collapse.

Reference

1. Wolfsdorf JI, Allgrove J, Craig ME, et al. ISPAD Clinical Practice Consensus Guidelines 2014. Diabetic ketoacidosis and hyperglycemic hyperosmolar state. *Pediatr Diabetes.* 2014;15 (Suppl 20):154–179.

CHAPTER 31

INTENSIVE INSULIN TREATMENT FOR TYPE 1 DIABETES

Mary Perry Alexander ■ Takara Stanley

The Effect of Intensive Treatment of Diabetes on the Development and Progression of Long-Term Complications in Insulin-Dependent Diabetes Mellitus

The Diabetes Control and Complications Trial (DCCT) Research Group. *N Engl J Med.* 1993;329(14):977–986

BACKGROUND

Many patients with type 1 diabetes mellitus (T1DM) develop severe complications such as retinopathy, nephropathy, neuropathy, and cardiovascular disease. In the late 1980s, it was not certain whether these complications were related to insulin use or hyperglycemia. This study sought to assess whether tighter glucose control reduced complications.

OBJECTIVES

To determine whether intensive insulin treatment for T1DM decreased the frequency and severity of complications such as retinopathy and nephropathy.

METHODS

Randomized controlled trial at 29 US centers from 1983 to 1989.

Patients

1,441 total patients ages 13 to 39 years with insulin-dependent T1DM: 726 primary-prevention patients with no retinopathy or nephropathy (albumin excretion ratio <40 mg/24 h) and 715 secondary-prevention patients with mild-to-moderate retinopathy and nephropathy (albumin excretion ratio <200 mg/24 h). Select exclusion criteria: hypertension, hypercholesterolemia, severe medical conditions.

Intervention

Intensive therapy (>3 insulin injections daily or an insulin pump combined with frequent blood glucose checks to achieve preprandial glucoses of 70 to 120 mg/dL and postprandial glucoses under 180 mg/dL, monthly examinations, and frequent phone contact) as compared to conventional therapy (1 to 2 daily insulin injections, examinations every 3 months). Participants were followed for an average of 6.5 years with a 99% study completion rate.

Outcomes

Primary outcome was development of clinically significant retinopathy. Secondary outcomes included development of nephropathy (microalbuminuria [≥40 mg/24 h] and albuminuria [≥300 mg/24 h]), neuropathy (abnormal neurologic examination) and macrovascular disease (hypercholesterolemia, cardiovascular events), and adverse effects.

KEY RESULTS

- Compared to conventional therapy, the primary-prevention group experienced reductions in the risk of retinopathy (76%, 95% CI 62–85), microalbuminuria (34%, 95% CI 2–56), and neuropathy (69%, 95% CI 24–87).
- Compared to conventional therapy, the secondary-prevention group experienced reductions in risk of retinopathy (54%, 95% CI 39–66), albuminuria (56%, 95% CI 18–76), and neuropathy (57%, 95% CI 29–73).
- Compared to the standard treatment group, the intensive therapy group had 3 times the incidence of severe hypoglycemia (62 vs. 19 events/100 patient-years).

STUDY CONCLUSIONS

Maintaining near-normal glucose levels through intensive insulin therapy in patients with T1DM slowed the development and progression of retinopathy, nephropathy, and neuropathy.

COMMENTARY

This landmark DCCT study established intensive insulin therapy as standard of care for T1DM, laying the groundwork for today's focus on targeting hemoglobin A1c (HbA1c) values. The overt clinical superiority of intensive treatment led to early discontinuation of the study. The authors noted, however, that intensive control of blood glucose was costly, required a multidisciplinary team, and increased the risk of severe hypoglycemia. The Epidemiology of Diabetes Interventions and Complications (EDIC) study, a long-term follow-up study of this DCCT cohort, demonstrated that intensive insulin therapy also reduced risk of cardiovascular events.[1] Interestingly, even though HbA1c values post-intervention were not different between groups in EDIC, reductions in T1DM complications persisted, suggesting that cumulative lifetime exposure to hyperglycemia is relevant.

Question

Can type 1 diabetes be effectively treated with 1 or 2 insulin injections daily?

Answer

No. Patients receiving only 1 or 2 daily injections of insulin (conventional therapy at the time of this study) went on to develop retinopathy, nephropathy, and neuropathy at a far greater rate than those on an insulin pump or 3 times daily injections, establishing today's standard of care of intensive glycemic control.

Reference

1. Nathan DM, Cleary PA, Backlund JY, et al. Intensive diabetes treatment and cardiovascular disease in patients with type 1 diabetes. *N Engl J Med.* 2005;353(25):2643–2653.

PREVENTION OF INTELLECTUAL IMPAIRMENT WITH NEONATAL HYPOTHYROIDISM SCREENING

Mary Perry Alexander ■ Takara Stanley

Effects of Neonatal Screening for Hypothyroidism: Prevention of Mental Retardation by Treatment Before Clinical Manifestations

New England Congenital Hypothyroidism Collaborative. *Lancet.* 1981;2(8255):1095–1098

BACKGROUND

Untreated congenital hypothyroidism (CH) is known to cause impaired intellectual development and neuropsychological problems. The advent of neonatal screening for hypothyroidism in the 1970s allowed infants with low thyroxine (T4) and elevated thyroid-stimulating hormone (TSH) to be identified and treated before any clinical evidence of hypothyroidism was apparent. This study presented the intelligence quotient (IQ) outcomes for a cohort of infants found to be hypothyroid on newborn screening at a time when newborn screening programs were in their infancy.

OBJECTIVES

To determine the impact of early thyroid hormone replacement on the intellectual development of infants identified as hypothyroid on routine newborn screening.

METHODS

Retrospective, case-control study in 5 US states from 1976 to 1978.

Patients

77 infants with hypothyroidism (T4 level <6 mcg/dL and TSH concentration >40 µU/dL on 2 blood tests, or between 20 to 40 µU/dL on 3 to 4 tests) diagnosed by routine screening of over 300,000 infants, and 4 infants diagnosed clinically at birth. Control group was 18 normal siblings and 39 euthyroid infants with low T4 but normal TSH.

Intervention

Infants found to be hypothyroid on newborn screening were treated with levothyroxine, and their development and IQ at ages 1–2 and 3–4 years were compared to the IQs of control group of normal siblings and euthyroid infants, as well as the infants with clinically diagnosed hypothyroidism.

Outcomes

Primary outcome was mean IQ as determined by the revised Stanford–Binet scales.

KEY RESULTS

- Mean IQ score at 3 to 4 years of 63 infants treated for screening-diagnosed hypo-thyroidism was 106 ± 16, essentially identical to the mean IQ of 106 ± 15 of the 57 controls.
- 3/4 infants with overt hypothyroidism at birth had low IQs (50, 64, 76) despite early treatment with levothyroxine.

STUDY CONCLUSIONS

Neonates treated with levothyroxine for subclinical CH identified by newborn screening attained normal IQs comparable to controls, whereas infants who were treated after the development of clinical features had low IQs in early childhood.

COMMENTARY

These results resoundingly supported a newborn screening program to diagnose CH and allow for early levothyroxine treatment. This screening represents a major achievement of preventive medicine, rescuing approximately 1:3,000 infants born with CH in developed countries from a lifetime of neurologic impairment. Newborns either have a primary TSH screen or a primary free T4 screen, with subsequent TSH testing for those with relatively lower T4 values; both have relative merits. Primary TSH screening is highly sensitive for primary CH but may miss secondary CH (due to pituitary insufficiency), whereas the primary T4 strategy may miss mild cases of primary CH but could pick up secondary CH. Newborn screening should be performed >24 hours of life, and ideally between 48 and 72 hours, to reduce false positives from the expected perinatal TSH surge. Of note, special screening strategies are recommended for premature infants.[1] Unfortunately, many developing nations still lack newborn screening, and infants in these countries are not identified and treated until they develop clinical symptoms, at which point treatment fails to preserve the child's intellectual potential.

Question

Does CH always result in intellectual impairment?

Answer

No. Asymptomatic infants who are identified as hypothyroid on newborn screen and have rapid initiation of treatment can be effectively treated with thyroid hormone replacement and go on to reach normal intellectual ability.

Reference

1. Léger J, Olivieri A, Donaldson M, et al. European Society for Paediatric Endocrinology consensus guide-lines on screening, diagnosis, and management of congenital hypothyroidism. *J Clin Endocrinol Metab.* 2014;99(2):363–384.

GASTROENTEROLOGY

6

33. Introduction of Gluten and Celiac Disease Risk
34. Use of PUCAI Score in Ulcerative Colitis
35. Infliximab Therapy for Crohn's Disease
36. Prevalence of Celiac Disease
37. Polyethylene Glycol Treatment for Constipation

INTRODUCTION OF GLUTEN AND CELIAC DISEASE RISK

Kathryn E. Wynne ■ Christopher J. Moran

Introduction of Gluten, HLA Status, and the Risk of Celiac Disease in Children
Lionetti E, Castellaneta S, Francavilla R, et al. *N Engl J Med.* 2014;371(14):1295–1303

BACKGROUND

Celiac disease (CD) is an autoimmune enteritis caused by gluten ingestion. It affects up to 3.5% of those with GI symptoms or a positive family history.[1] Genetic susceptibility plays a strong role as nearly all patients with CD carry a high-risk HLA allele (HLA-DQ2 or HLA-DQ8). Prior studies suggested a window of tolerance between 4 to 6 months of age, during which infants may achieve immune tolerance through early gluten introduction due to potential protective effects of breastfeeding.[2,3] Some groups suggested gluten introduction during this period while others avoided making specific recommendations. This trial investigated the impact of timing of gluten introduction on CD development.

OBJECTIVES

To determine the relationship between age of gluten introduction and risk of CD in genetically susceptible infants.

METHODS

Randomized trial at 20 centers in Italy between 2003 and 2008.

Patients

553 newborns with ≥1 first-degree relatives with CD and high-risk HLA genotype (HLA-DQ2 or HLA-DQ8).

Intervention

Randomization to gluten introduction at age 6 (Group A) or 12 (Group B) months. CD serologies (including antitransglutaminase type 2 Immunoglobulin A) were sent at 15 months and 2, 3, 5, 8, and 10 years. Duodenal biopsy was recommended for positive serology. Patients were followed for ≥5 years.

Outcomes

Primary outcomes were prevalence of CD autoimmunity (CDA; positive serology) and overt CD (positive serology and biopsy) at age 5. Secondary outcomes included prevalence of CDA and overt CD at age 10, and effects of HLA genotype and breastfeeding.

KEY RESULTS
- Group A had more frequent CDA and CD compared to Group B (16% vs. 7%, $p = 0.002$ and 12% vs. 5%, $p = 0.01$) at age 2.
- There was no difference in CDA or CD between Groups A and B by age 5 (21% vs. 20%, $p = 0.59$).
- Median age of CD diagnosis was 26 months in Group A and 34 months in Group B ($p = 0.01$).
- At age 10, children with high-risk HLA genotype were more likely than those with standard-risk HLA genotype to have CDA (38% vs. 19%, $p = 0.001$) or CD (26% vs. 16%, $p = 0.05$) regardless of timing of gluten introduction.
- Breastfeeding rates at the time of gluten introduction were similar between children who developed CD and those who did not (20.4% vs. 20.0%).

STUDY CONCLUSIONS
CD prevalence was not affected by timing of gluten introduction in genetically susceptible infants but later introduction did delay CD onset. HLA genotype was associated with CD risk, whereas breastfeeding was not.

COMMENTARY
Although delayed gluten introduction did not prevent CD, it may be beneficial in high-risk infants by postponing CD onset and sequelae until after the period of early childhood development. As this study had minimal subject diversity and a higher drop-out rate in those with delayed gluten introduction, future research is needed to assess other potential interventions that may prevent CD in high-risk children.

Question
Does delayed gluten introduction (>12 months of age) reduce risk of CD?

Answer
No. However, delaying gluten introduction can delay disease onset, offering potential benefit during early childhood growth and development.

References
1. Fasano A, Berti I, Gerarduzzi T, et al. Prevalence of celiac disease in at-risk and not-at-risk groups in the United States: A large multicenter study. *Arch Intern Med.* 2003;163(3):286–292.
2. Norris JM, Barriga K, Hoffenberg EJ, et al. Risk of celiac disease autoimmunity and timing of gluten introduction in the diet of infants at increased risk of disease. *JAMA.* 2005;293(19):2343–2351.
3. Ivarsson A, Myléus A, Norström F, et al. Prevalence of childhood celiac disease and changes in infant feeding. *Pediatrics.* 2013;131(3):e687–e694.

CHAPTER 34

USE OF PUCAI SCORE IN ULCERATIVE COLITIS

Kathryn E. Wynne ■ Christopher J. Moran

Severe Pediatric Ulcerative Colitis: A Prospective Multicenter Study of Outcomes and Predictors of Response

Turner D, Mack D, Leleiko N, et al. *Gastroenterology.* 2010;138(7):2282–2291

BACKGROUND

Children with ulcerative colitis (UC) present with more extensive inflammation than adults, increasing their risk for severe exacerbations.[1] Nearly half of children admitted with exacerbations are corticosteroid refractory and require salvage therapy (including cyclosporine, infliximab, and/or colectomy).[2] Corticosteroid-refractory disease must therefore be identified quickly to limit complications and adverse medication effects. The Pediatric UC Activity Index (PUCAI) was developed to assess overall disease severity based on pain, rectal bleeding, activity level, stool consistency and frequency, and nocturnal stooling. A score of <10 is remission, 10 to 34 is mild, 35 to 64 is moderate, and 65 to 85 is severe disease.[3] This study assessed the utility of the PUCAI to predict steroid-refractory UC.

OBJECTIVES

To identify early predictors of steroid-refractory UC in children.

METHODS

Prospective, longitudinal, observational study at 10 centers in the US, Canada, Israel, and Australia from 2006 to 2008.

Patients

128 children ages 2 to 18 years diagnosed with UC exacerbation who were admitted for IV corticosteroids (IVCS). Select exclusion criteria: limited proctitis, enteric infection, history of biologic therapy.

Intervention

Children were managed by their primary gastroenterologist. Data were collected on days 1, 3, and 5 of IVCS therapy, upon salvage therapy introduction (if used), and upon discharge including: PUCAI, 3 adult-based severity indices, laboratory markers (complete blood count, albumin, erythrocyte sedimentation rate, and C-reactive protein), medications, and nutritional status. Follow-up data were collected at 12 months.

Outcomes

Primary outcome was short-term response to IVCS. Secondary outcome was response to salvage therapy.

KEY RESULTS

- 29% of children did not respond to IVCS therapy (95% CI 22–37).
- PUCAI was the strongest predictor of response compared to other measures ($p < 0.001$).
- PUCAI >45 on day 3 or >70 on day 5 were highly predictive for identifying children likely to fail IVCS therapy (NPV 94%, PPV 43%, and NPV 79%, PPV 100%, respectively, $p < 0.001$).
- 89% of children who did not respond to IVCS received infliximab as salvage therapy. 76% had an initial response, and 55% of those had a sustained response at 1 year.

STUDY CONCLUSIONS

PUCAI scores at days 3 and 5 identified children likely to require salvage therapy. Infliximab proved effective in steroid-refractory UC.

COMMENTARY

Although the PUCAI was developed to assess overall disease severity, this study demonstrated its application as a short-term predictive index in severe pediatric UC flares. The high NPV of the day 3 PUCAI identified most steroid nonresponders. A limitation is that treating physicians were not blinded to the PUCAI scores which may have contributed to escalation of therapy. Infliximab was commonly used for salvage therapy during the study period and was confirmed efficacious in this population. This study prompted pediatric UC treatment guidelines to recommend routine calculation of PUCAI in hospitalized children.[2]

Question

Can we predict which children with severe UC receiving IVCS therapy will need salvage therapy?

Answer

Yes. The PUCAI score can be used which is timely, easy to calculate, and the most accurate marker to predict steroid nonresponse and need to escalate therapy.

References

1. Turner D, Levine A, Escher JC, et al. Management of pediatric ulcerative colitis: Joint ECCO and ESP-GHAN evidence-based consensus guidelines. *J Pediatr Gastroenterol Nutr.* 2012;55(3):340–361.
2. Turner D, Walsh CM, Benchimol EI, et al. Severe paediatric ulcerative colitis: Incidence, outcomes and optimal timing for second-line therapy. *Gut.* 2008;57(3):331–338.
3. Turner D, Otley AR, Mack D, et al. Development, validation, and evaluation of a pediatric ulcerative colitis activity index: A prospective multicenter study. *Gastroenterology.* 2007;133(2):423–432.

CHAPTER 35

INFLIXIMAB THERAPY FOR CROHN'S DISEASE

Kathryn E. Wynne ■ Christopher J. Moran

Induction and Maintenance Infliximab Therapy for the Treatment of Moderate-to-Severe Crohn's Disease in Children (The Reach Trial)

Hyams J, Crandall W, Kugathasan S, et al. *Gastroenterology.* 2007;132(3):863–873

BACKGROUND

For children with Crohn's disease (CD) who fail conventional therapy (5-aminosalicy-lates, immunomodulators), few treatment options were previously available. Infliximab is a monoclonal antibody against tumor necrosis factor-α (TNF-α) that became available for adults with CD in 1998 after clinical trials showed efficacy as salvage therapy.[1] However, until this study, infliximab had not been rigorously studied in pediatric CD and there were concerns about tumor and infection risk.

OBJECTIVES

To assess the efficacy of induction and maintenance regimens with infliximab for pediatric CD.

METHODS

Randomized, open-label study at 34 sites in North America, Europe, and Israel from 2003 to 2004.

Patients

112 children ages 6 to 17 years with moderate-to-severe CD (Pediatric Crohn's Disease Activity Index [PCDAI] >30 at baseline) on stable immunomodulator dosing. Select exclusion criterion: prior treatment with anti–TNF-α agents.

Intervention

Patients underwent induction with infliximab 5 mg/kg at weeks 0, 2, and 6. Patients with response at week 10 (PCDAI ≤30 with decrease of ≥15) were randomized to maintenance therapy with infliximab every 8 or 12 weeks. Dose escalation was allowed once for waning clinical response.

Outcomes

Primary outcomes were rates of clinical response/remission after induction and mainte-nance therapy. Clinical remission was defined as PCDAI ≤10. Secondary outcome was number of patients requiring maintenance intensification and adverse events.

KEY RESULTS

- 88.4% of patients responded to infliximab induction at week 10 (95% CI 82.5–94.3), with 58.9% in clinical remission (95% CI 49.8–68).
- At week 54, the patients receiving infliximab every 8 weeks had higher rates of clinical response (63.5% vs. 33.3%, $p = 0.002$) and remission (55.8% vs. 23.5%, $p < 0.001$) than patients receiving infliximab every 12 weeks.
- Only 19.2% of patients receiving maintenance infliximab every 8 weeks required dosing intensification vs. 49% in the every-12-week group.
- Adverse events occurred more frequently among patients receiving infliximab every 8 weeks as opposed to every 12 weeks (73.6% vs. 38%), though incidence of serious infection was similar (5.7% vs. 8%).

STUDY CONCLUSIONS

Infliximab induction therapy was effective in pediatric CD. Rates of clinical response and remission at week 54 were superior in the every-8-week regimen compared to the every-12-week regimen.

COMMENTARY

This study demonstrated the superior efficacy of more frequent (every-8-week) infliximab maintenance therapy. Of note, patients received stable, concomitant immunomodulator therapy and were anti–TNFα-naïve, which may limit the study's generalizability. These results were instrumental in the development of clinical guidelines for pediatric CD therapy.[2] Infliximab-related adverse events, including infection and lymphoma, are a significant concern. This study found a reassuringly low serious infection rate, though it was not powered for assessment of lymphoma risk. Furthermore, a subsequent meta-analysis showed that infliximab did not increase the risk of serious infections or lymphoma in children with IBD.[3]

Question

Is infliximab an effective treatment for pediatric CD?

Answer

Yes. In this study, induction with infliximab 5 mg/kg followed by maintenance dosing every 8 weeks was most effective in inducing clinical response and remission.

References

1. Hanauer SB, Feagan BG, Lichtenstein GR, et al. Maintenance infliximab for Crohn's disease: The ACCENT I randomised trial. *Lancet.* 2002;359(9317):1541–1549.
2. Ruemmele FM, Veres G, Kolho KL, et al. Consensus guidelines of ECCO/ESPGHAN on the medical management of pediatric Crohn's disease. *J Crohns Colitis.* 2014;8(10):1179–1207.
3. Dulai PS, Thompson KD, Blunt HB, et al. Risks of serious infection or lymphoma with anti-tumor necrosis factor therapy for pediatric inflammatory bowel disease: A systematic review. *Clin Gastroenterol Hepatol.* 2014;12(9):1443–1451.

CHAPTER 36

PREVALENCE OF CELIAC DISEASE

Kathryn E. Wynne ■ Christopher J. Moran

Prevalence of Celiac Disease in At-Risk and Not-At-Risk Groups in the US: A Large Multicenter Study

Fasano A, Berti I, Gerarduzzi T, et al. *Arch Intern Med.* 2003;163(3):286–292

BACKGROUND

Though celiac disease (CD) was once thought to be a rare condition, the prevalence of the diagnosis in European populations increased markedly from 1:4,000 to 1:340 from 1970 to 1990.[1,2] It is now recognized that the classic symptoms of diarrhea, abdominal pain, and weight loss do not encompass all disease presentations. This was the first large-scale study to evaluate the prevalence of CD in the US.

OBJECTIVES

To determine the prevalence of CD in at-risk and not-at-risk groups in the US.

METHODS

Cross-sectional screening study in 32 US states from 1996 to 2001.

Patients

13,145 adults (ages 19 to 71 years) and children (ages 2 to 18 years): 9,019 at-risk subjects (first- and second-degree relatives with CD, or CD-associated symptoms/ disorders) and 4,126 not-at-risk subjects. Select exclusion criteria: none.

Intervention

Patients had serum anti-gliadin antibodies and anti-endomysial antibodies (anti-EMA) measured. If they were EMA positive, further testing was obtained (tissue transglutaminase Immunoglobulin A antibody [TTG IgA], CD-associated HLA DQ2/DQ8 haplotype, and intestinal biopsy). A diagnosis of CD was made when a patient had a positive EMA and either a duodenal biopsy consistent with CD or HLA haplotype sufficient for CD (if no biopsy performed).

Outcomes

Primary outcome measure was prevalence of CD in at-risk and not-at-risk patients.

KEY RESULTS

- CD prevalence in at-risk patients was 4.55% (95% CI 3.9) in those with first-degree relatives with CD, 2.59% (95% CI 1.8–3.6) in those with second-degree relatives

with CD, 1.47% (95% CI 0.97–2.1) in symptomatic adults, and 4% (95% CI 2.99–5.2) in symptomatic children.
- CD prevalence in not-at-risk patients was 0.95% (95% CI 0.6–1.4) in adults and 0.31% (95% CI 0.09–0.8) in children.
- All 350 EMA-positive subjects were TTG IgA-positive and had HLA haplotypes consistent with CD.

STUDY CONCLUSIONS
The prevalence of CD in the US was much higher than that had been previously suspected.

COMMENTARY

CD is much more common in the US than previously believed, particularly in individuals with a genetic predisposition. Of note, only 33% of EMA-positive subjects underwent biopsy, which remains the gold standard for CD diagnosis. In addition, minority groups made up only 6% of the study population; further studies are needed to determine the prevalence in these groups. This study significantly influenced CD clinical guidelines by expanding screening recommendations to include children and adults with first-degree relatives with CD, those with CD-associated nongastrointestinal symptoms (osteoporosis, short stature, and unexplained anemia), and those with CD-associated conditions (trisomy 21, Williams syndrome, and diabetes mellitus).[3]

Question

How prevalent is CD in the US?

Answer

Prevalence ranges from 0.75% in asymptomatic adults and children without family history of CD to 3.54% in adults and children with suggestive symptoms or family history of CD. Given the increased prevalence in these at-risk groups, screening is recommended for people with a family history of CD (in a first-degree family member) in addition to those with symptoms suggestive of CD.

References
1. Kolho KL, Färkkilä MA, Savilahti E. Undiagnosed coeliac disease is common in Finnish adults. *Scand J Gastroenterol.* 1998;33(12):1280–1283.
2. Ascher H, Krantz I, Kristiansson B. Increasing incidence of coeliac disease in Sweden. *Arch Dis Child.* 1991;66(5):608–611.
3. Hill ID, Dirks MH, Liptak GS. Guideline for the diagnosis and treatment of celiac disease in children: Recommendations of the North American Society for Pediatric Gastroenterology, Hepatology, and Nutrition. *J Pediatr Gastroenterol Nutr.* 2005;40(1):1–19.

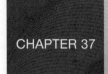

POLYETHYLENE GLYCOL TREATMENT FOR CONSTIPATION

CHAPTER 37

Kathryn E. Wynne ■ Christopher J. Moran

Efficacy and Optimal Dose of Daily Polyethylene Glycol 3350 for Treatment of Constipation and Encopresis in Children

Pashankar DS, Bishop WP. *J Pediatr*. 2001;139(3):428–432

BACKGROUND
Constipation occurs in 3% of children.[1] While treatment options for chronic constipation are numerous, they often have unpleasant tastes that prevent long-term compliance, particularly in children.[2] Polyethylene glycol 3350 (PEG), an osmotic agent, had been shown to be safe and efficacious for constipation in adults in the 1990s; only preliminary reports were available on use in pediatrics.

OBJECTIVES
To determine the efficacy, safety, and optimal dose of PEG in children with chronic constipation.

METHODS
Prospective, noncontrolled, open-label trial at a single US academic center.

Patients
24 children ages 18 months to 11 years with a diagnosis of chronic constipation (>3 months of two of the following: hard stools, painful stooling, stool withholding, fecal soiling, palpable stool mass, and <3 bowel movements per week). Select exclusion criteria: Hirschsprung disease, anorectal malformation, abdominal surgery, or systemic illness causing constipation.

Intervention
PEG was initiated at a dose of 1 g/kg/d (divided twice daily) for 8 weeks; other medications for constipation were discontinued. Parents adjusted the PEG dose by 20% every 3 days as needed to result in 2 soft-to-loose stools daily. Parents documented stool frequency, consistency (on scale from 1 = hard to 5 = watery), soiling frequency, associated symptoms, dose given, and any adverse effects daily.

Outcomes
Primary outcomes were patient compliance, stool frequency and consistency, frequency of soiling, and optimal PEG dose.

KEY RESULTS
- 4 children were excluded from analyses due to excessive stooling. All children who completed the study found PEG to be palatable and effective. No patient stopped treatment because of adverse effects.
- Weekly stool frequency increased from 2.3 ± 0.4 to 16.9 ± 1.6 ($p < 0.0001$).
- Stool consistency improved from 1.2 ± 0.1 to 3.3 ± 0.1 ($p < 0.0001$).
- For the 9 patients with encopresis, weekly frequency of soiling declined from 10 ± 2.4 to 1.3 ± 0.7 ($p = 0.003$).
- Mean effective dose was 0.84 g/kg/d (range 0.27–1.42 g/kg/d).

STUDY CONCLUSIONS
PEG administered at a dose of 0.8 g/kg/d was an effective, safe, and palatable treatment for children with constipation.

COMMENTARY
PEG was introduced as a prescription-only drug in 1999 with an emphasis on its palatability. While this study was the first to establish its safety and efficacy in children, there were significant drawbacks: small size, short duration, lack of blinding or control group, and reliance on parents for symptom assessments and medication dose adjustments. However, subsequent studies have supported these data, showing PEG to be more effective than lactulose in children with constipation.[2] PEG is now a first-line treatment for pediatric constipation.[3] More recently, potential neuropsychiatric effects have been reported to the Food and Drug Administration. Large-scale, longitudinal studies are needed to evaluate the long-term safety of PEG.

Question
Can PEG be used in treatment of children with constipation?

Answer
Yes. PEG proved safe and effective at a dose of 0.8 g/kg/d divided twice daily, and is now first-line constipation therapy in children.

References
1. van den Berg MM, Benninga MA, Di Lorenzo C. Epidemiology of childhood constipation: A systematic review. *Am J Gastroenterol.* 2006;101(10):2401–2409.
2. Lee-Robichaud H, Thomas K, Morgan J, et al. Lactulose versus Polyethylene Glycol for Chronic Constipation. *Cochrane Database Syst Rev.* 2010;(7):CD007570.
3. Tabbers MM, DiLorenzo C, Berger MY, et al. Evaluation and treatment of functional constipation in infants and children: Evidence-based recommendations from ESPGHAN and NASPGHAN. *J Pediatr Gastroenterol Nutr.* 2014;58(2):258–274.

GENETICS

38. Whole-Exome Sequencing
39. Noninvasive Prenatal Testing for Trisomy 21
40. Mass Spectrometry Screening for Inborn Errors of Metabolism
41. Angiotensin Receptor Blockade in Marfan Syndrome

CHAPTER 38

WHOLE-EXOME SEQUENCING

Lila Worden ■ David A. Sweetser

Clinical Whole-Exome Sequencing for the Diagnosis of Mendelian Disorders
Yang Y, Muzny DM, Reid JG, et al. *N Engl J Med.* 2013;369(16):1502–1511

BACKGROUND

Worldwide, recognized genetic disorders occur in 40 to 82 per 1,000 live births.[1] The majority of patients who present to a genetic clinic, however, do not receive a molecular diagnosis despite lengthy and expensive evaluations, limiting access to appropriate counseling and support. With the advent of whole-exome sequencing (WES), all 23,000 genes can now be sequenced in a single test. Since its availability in 2011, numerous published case reports had cited benefit in patients with previously undiagnosed conditions, but the value of WES in wider clinical practice remained unknown.

OBJECTIVES

To measure the diagnostic yield of WES in patients referred for evaluation of a possible genetic condition.

METHODS

Consecutive case series at a single US academic center from 2011 to 2012.

Patients

250 patient samples (4 fetal, 218 pediatric, 28 adult) from individuals with prior genetic workups referred for WES. Select exclusion criteria: none.

Intervention

WES, with expert review of records and application of rigorous algorithms to interpret whether variants were pathogenic. Clinically significant variants were confirmed by traditional sequencing methods and parental samples were sequenced when available.

Outcomes

Primary outcome was diagnostic yield of patient samples. Secondary outcome was rate of unrelated secondary findings warranting medical action.

KEY RESULTS

- Reason for performance of WES was primarily neurologic, including developmental delay, autism, or movement disorders (85%).
- Positive genetic diagnoses were found in 62/250 cases (25%, 95% CI 20–31).

- Diagnostic yield was best for neurologic disorder phenotypes, both nonspecific and specific (33%, 95% CI 23–46 and 31%, 95% CI 13–58, respectively).
- 30/250 (12%) had medically significant secondary findings, including carrier mutations, cancer susceptibility genes, and genes affecting drug metabolism.

STUDY CONCLUSIONS

WES was a useful diagnostic test for patients with unusual clinical presentations of a possible genetic etiology, or with clinical diagnoses with multiple genetic causes for which specific testing was unavailable.

COMMENTARY

This study was the first to demonstrate that WES had a diagnostic yield of 25% in cases with prior extensive negative testing, which is notable compared to the general diagnostic yield of other genetic tests: 5% to 15% for karyotyping, 15% to 20% for chromosomal microarray, and 3% to 40% for single gene panels. The relatively impressive diagnostic yield of WES has since been confirmed in a larger study of 2,000 patients.[2] The overall utility of the test, however, is currently limited by extremely high cost and limited insurance coverage, incomplete knowledge of gene functions, detection of nonpathologic sequence variants, and poor identification of duplications and deletions. The American College of Medical Genetics recommends considering WES when there is strong evidence for a genetic etiology but a phenotype-driven targeted gene search is not possible, or in cases where available testing has been unsuccessful.[3] The complexity of this test requires extensive pre- and post-test counseling by a specialist with appropriate genetic expertise.

Question

When should you consider WES in the evaluation of a possible genetic disorder?

Answer

WES has a comparable diagnostic yield to the best currently available tests, but given current limitations, chromosomal microarray or targeted gene testing are still first line if appropriate.

References

1. Christianson AL, Howson CP, Modell B. *March of Dimes Global Report on Birth Defects: The Hidden Toll of Dying and Disabled Children.* White Plains, NY: March of Dimes Birth Defects Foundation, 2006. http://www.marchofdimes.org/materials/global-report-on-birth-defects-the-hidden-toll-of-dying-and-disabled-children-executive-summary.pdf. Accessed on July 20, 2015.
2. Yang Y, Muzny DM, Xia F, et al. Molecular findings among patients referred for clinical whole-exome sequencing. *JAMA.* 2014;312(18):1870–1879.
3. ACMG Board of Directors. Points to consider in the clinical application of genomic sequencing. *Genet Med.* 2012;14(8):759–761.

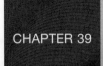

CHAPTER 39 — NONINVASIVE PRENATAL TESTING FOR TRISOMY 21

Lila Worden ■ David A. Sweetser

Non-Invasive Prenatal Assessment of Trisomy 21 by Multiplexed Maternal Plasma DNA Sequencing: Large Scale Validity Study

Chiu RW, Akolekar R, Zheng YW, et al. *BMJ.* 2011;342:c7401

BACKGROUND

Trisomy 21 (T21) is the most common chromosomal abnormality, affecting 1:800 live births. Despite increased use of ultrasonography and serum biomarker screening for T21, invasive testing (chorionic villus sampling [CVS] or amniocentesis) is still required in 3% to 5% of patients and has a miscarriage risk of approximately 1%.[1] In 1997, cell-free DNA (cfDNA) fragments from the fetus were discovered in maternal plasma but in a relatively small proportion, limiting clinical use.[2] The advent of massively parallel sequencing (MPS) technology enabled amplification of cfDNA, but application of this method for T21 screening had only been demonstrated in small cohort studies previously.

OBJECTIVES

To determine the accuracy and feasibility of MPS of maternal DNA for use in prenatal screening for T21 in high-risk pregnancies.

METHODS

Review of archived samples from T21 cases (2003 to 2008) matched 1:5 with controls and prospectively recruited high-risk pregnant women (2008 to 2009) at 10 sites across Hong Kong, the Netherlands, and the United Kingdom.

Patients

753 plasma samples from 824 singleton pregnancies with clinical indication for CVS or amniocentesis. Select exclusion criteria: full karyotype unavailable, poor specimen or sequencing quality.

Intervention

MPS of maternal plasma analyzed via 8-plex processing with subsequent 2-plex processing (co-sequencing of 8 or 2 samples together) of positive cases and a subset of controls as compared to the gold standard of full karyotyping from amniocentesis or CVS.

Outcomes

Primary outcome was the number of samples with z-scores for chromosome 21 greater than 3 (i.e., T21). Secondary outcomes were test characteristics of the 2-plex versus 8-plex sequencing protocols.

KEY RESULTS

- Of 753 samples sequenced, 86 had T21, 40 had trisomy 18, 20 had trisomy 13, 8 had Turner syndrome, and 2 had sex chromosome mosaicism.
- 2-plex processing was superior to 8-plex in detecting T21 (100% sensitivity and 98% specificity vs. 79% and 99%, respectively) with better PPV (97% vs. 92%) and NPV (100% vs. 97%).
- False-positive rates were slightly higher with 2-plex sequencing (2.1% vs. 1.1%).

STUDY CONCLUSIONS

2-plex MPS of maternal DNA had high sensitivity and specificity for prenatal T21 diagnosis, reducing need for invasive testing by 98%.

COMMENTARY

This study was fundamental in the clinical adoption of cfDNA screening, demonstrating excellent diagnostic parameters and large-scale feasibility. Since 2011, it has been widely adopted in prenatal screening in high-risk pregnancies, and is moving toward use in all pregnancies. A recent prospective study of almost 19,000 pregnancies showed 100% sensitivity for T21 detection and a 0.06% false-positive rate, though cost-effectiveness for the general population remains unknown.[3] Limitations included need for amniocentesis or CVS for confirmation of positive tests. Nonetheless, cfDNA technology is only expanding: in addition to testing for other trisomies, there is increasing capability for detection of other sex chromosome aneuploidies and microdeletions.

Question

Is MPS of maternal DNA a valid prenatal screening test for T21?

Answer

Yes, it has 100% sensitivity and 98% specificity for detection of T21 and should be offered as a screen to rule out T21 as it decreases need for invasive procedures.

References

1. Kagan KO, Wright D, Baker A, et al. Screening for trisomy 21 by maternal age, fetal nuchal translucency thickness, free beta-human chorionic gonadotropin and pregnancy-associated plasma protein-A. *Ultrasound Obstet Gynecol.* 2008;31(6):618–624.
2. Lo YM, Corbetta N, Chamberlain PF, et al. Presence of fetal DNA in maternal plasma and serum. *Lancet.* 1997;350(9076):485–487.
3. Norton ME, Jacobsson B, Swamy GK, et al. Cell-free DNA analysis for noninvasive examination of trisomy. *N Engl J Med.* 2015;372(17):1589–1597.

CHAPTER 40

MASS SPECTROMETRY SCREENING FOR INBORN ERRORS OF METABOLISM

Lila Worden ■ David A. Sweetser

Diagnosis of Inborn Errors of Metabolism From Blood Spots by Acylcarnitines and Amino Acids Profiling Using Automated Electrospray Tandem Mass Spectrometry

Rashed MS, Ozand PT, Bucknall MP, et al. *Pediatr Res.* 1995;38(3):324–331

BACKGROUND

Since the 1960s, newborn screening (NBS) for early detection of metabolic disorders has helped prevent significant morbidity and mortality through early treatment. In the early 1990s, only a few inborn errors of metabolism (IEM), such as organic acidemias and amino acid catabolism disorders, could be screened for, and these required time- and labor-intensive single-enzyme assays. Tandem Mass Spectrometry (TMS), developed in 1990, had the potential to greatly expand NBS through the generation of acylcarnitine and amino acid biochemical profiles from fragmented ion samples of blood spots, allowing for simultaneous screening for multiple conditions. Prior small studies showed success using TMS to diagnose IEMs but the manual process remained labor intensive and potentially error prone. This study was the first to test the feasibility of automation and analysis with a large number of samples.

OBJECTIVES

To assess feasibility of large-scale TMS with simultaneous acylcarnitine and amino acid profiling and to determine accuracy of automation of the sample input.

METHODS

Qualitative study at a single metabolism center in Saudi Arabia over a 9-month period from 1993 to 1994.

Patients

Approximately 2,000 NBS samples, most with unknown diagnoses. Select exclusion criteria: none.

Intervention

Use of TMS technology to quantify and profile acylcarnitines and amino acids simultaneously, with an automation protocol for processing multiple specimens. Abnormal spectrometry profiles were confirmed by urine or blood tests when available.

Outcomes

Primary outcome was the determination of biochemical profiles of IEM cases. Secondary outcome was reliability of large-scale automation.

KEY RESULTS
- 52 new cases of IEM were diagnosed and 75 known cases were confirmed.
- Unique acylcarnitine and amino acid profiles were established for 14 different IEMs including fatty acid oxidation defects, branched-chain amino acid disorders, amino acid disorders, and urea cycle disorders.
- Automation with simultaneous acylcarnitine/amino acid profiling was possible without signal contamination carry-over (and take out parentheses as per edit) from 20 successive samples (15 abnormal, 5 normal).

STUDY CONCLUSIONS
TMS could be used in detection of a broad range of IEM using process automation without loss of test accuracy.

COMMENTARY
This study showed that TMS remained accurate and practical, even with large-scale automation, which was crucial in transforming this from a research tool to a population screening tool now widely used in NBS. This technology revolutionized NBS dramatically. In 2003, only 4 US states screened for >6 disorders; now all states screen for at least 29 core disorders recommended for universal screening by the American College of Medical Genetics.[1,2] Given the lack of federal mandate and varied resource allocation, state-by-state variability can be significant, with some states screening as many as 60 disorders. Now, with an additional 3,400 infants diagnosed each year with 1 of the 29 core disorders, expansion of NBS with adoption of TMS remains one of the great public health achievements.[1]

Question
Is automated TMS specific and accurate in the diagnosis of organic acidemias and amino acid disorders via NBS?

Answer
Yes, automation allows for expanded screening with a small blood sample yet retains high accuracy, allowing for its use in large populations as required for NBS.

References
1. Centers for Disease Control and Prevention (CDC). Ten great public health achievements—United States, 2001-2010. *MMWR Morb Mortal Wkly Rep.* 2011;60(19):619–623.
2. American College of Medical Genetics Newborn Screening Expert Group. Newborn screening: Toward a uniform screening panel and system—executive summary. *Pediatrics.* 2006;117(5 Pt 2):S296–S307.

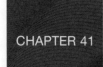

ANGIOTENSIN RECEPTOR BLOCKADE IN MARFAN SYNDROME

CHAPTER 41

Lila Worden ■ David A. Sweetser

Angiotensin II Blockade and Aortic-Root Dilation in Marfan's Syndrome

Brooke BS, Habashi JP, Judge DP, et al. *N Engl J Med.* 2008;358(26):2787–2795

BACKGROUND

Aortic dissection is the leading cause of premature death in patients with Marfan syndrome, a connective tissue disorder caused by a fibrillin gene mutation affecting 1:5,000 people. Beta-blockers (BB) are used to reduce the rate of aortic dilation, delaying need for surgical intervention. Mouse models demonstrated that excess transforming growth factor-β (TGF-β) underlies the pathologic aortic changes. TGF-β blockade with angiotensin II receptor blockers (ARB) had been shown to reduce aortic dilation in mice, but evidence in humans was absent.[1]

OBJECTIVES

To evaluate the effect of ARBs on rate of progression of aortic dilation in patients with Marfan syndrome.

METHODS

Retrospective cohort study at a single US center from 1996 to 2007.

Patients

18 patients ages 14 months to 16 years with severe Marfan syndrome who were started on ARB based on intolerance of other agents or clinical need (rapid rate of dilation or severe aortic root enlargement). 65 patients on BB monotherapy with mild aortic dilation served as controls. Select exclusion criteria: medication nonadherence.

Intervention

Administration of losartan (17/18 patients, titrated to 1.4 mg/kg/d) or irbesartan (1/18 patients, titrated to 2 mg/kg/d) with continuation of BB for >1 year. Angiotensin converting enzyme inhibitors and calcium channel blockers were discontinued. Rate of aortic dilation was compared pre- versus post-ARB initiation as well as to controls. Patients had echocardiograms every 3 to 12 months.

Outcomes

Primary outcomes were both absolute and relative change in aortic root diameter (z-score normalized to body surface area and age). Secondary outcomes were changes in other aortic measurements and tolerability (heart rate, blood pressure, and renal function).

KEY RESULTS

- There was a significant decrease in the median absolute rate of aortic root dilation (0.3 mm/y vs. 3.3 mm/y, $p < 0.001$) and relative rate (−0.5 z-scores/y vs. 1.0 z-scores/y, $p < 0.001$) after ARB therapy as compared to before.
- Rate of dilation in controls was greater than those in intervention group post-ARB (0.1 z-scores/y vs. −0.5 z-scores/y, $p < 0.001$).
- There was a decline in height velocity post-ARB, with significant decreases in median height velocity z-scores (0.7 vs. −1.3, $p < 0.05$).
- No other adverse events occurred on ARB therapy.

STUDY CONCLUSIONS

In patients with severe Marfan syndrome, addition of ARB to BB was well tolerated and cohort data showed slowing of the rate of aortic root dilation.

COMMENTARY

The significant effect size in this study prompted most clinicians to change practice solely based on these results, routinely prescribing ARBs for patients with severe aortic dilation to try to prevent the need for cardiac surgery. Recently, the benefit of ARB therapy in Marfan has been questioned by a large prospective randomized trial comparing losartan vs. atenolol that did not find any significant difference in the rate of aortic dilation.[2] The results are controversial, however, as it evaluated ARB alone instead of in combination with BB, used high BB and low ARB doses, and studied an older cohort. Additional studies to evaluate the role of ARBs in Marfan are currently ongoing.

Question

Are ARBs useful in slowing progression of aortic dilation in patients with severe Marfan syndrome?

Answer

Maybe. Although this retrospective study showed strong benefit in combination with BBs, subsequent evidence showed no benefit alone, so additional studies are underway to determine whether they benefit specific patient subgroups.

References

1. Habashi JP, Judge DP, Holm TM, et al. Losartan, an AT1 antagonist, prevents aortic aneurysm in a mouse model of Marfan syndrome. *Science.* 2006;312(5770):117–121.
2. Lacro RV, Dietz HC, Sleeper LA, et al. Atenolol versus losartan in children and young adults with Marfan's syndrome. *N Engl J Med.* 2014;371(22):2061–2071.

HEMATOLOGY/ ONCOLOGY

42. Genetic Predictors of Unfavorable Outcomes in Pediatric Medulloblastoma
43. Prophylactic Treatment With Factor VIII in Hemophilia
44. Significance of Minimal Residual Disease in Acute Lymphoblastic Leukemia
45. Increased Incidence of Chronic Disease in Survivors of Childhood Cancers
46. Treatment of Acute Idiopathic Thrombocytopenic Purpura
47. Hydroxyurea Therapy in Sickle Cell Anemia
48. Symptom Management at the End of Life in Pediatric Oncology
49. Stroke Risk Reduction in Sickle Cell Anemia

GENETIC PREDICTORS OF UNFAVORABLE OUTCOMES IN PEDIATRIC MEDULLOBLASTOMA

Patricia A. Stoeck ■ Howard J. Weinstein

Outcome Prediction in Pediatric Medulloblastoma Based on DNA Copy-Number Aberrations of Chromosomes 6q and 17q and the MYC and MYCN Loci

Pfister S, Remke M, Benner A, et al. *J Clin Oncol.* 2009;27(10):1627–1636

BACKGROUND

Medulloblastoma is the most common pediatric brain tumor. Although 60% of these patients are ultimately cured, 10% to 15% die within 2 years of diagnosis and those who survive face significant adverse treatment effects. Previously, age, metastatic disease, and scope of surgical resection determined stratification into standard or high-risk grouping, but significant heterogeneity in outcomes was observed within groups. This study sought to identify chromosomal regions predictive of disease outcome to refine conventional staging methods.

OBJECTIVES

To incorporate specific genetic aberrations into a model for determining prognosis, including overall survival (OS) and progression-free survival (PFS), in pediatric medulloblastoma.

METHODS

Screening/validation study with screening tissue samples from Germany and Russia collected from 1994 to 2002 and validation samples from Russia collected from 1995 to 2006.

Patients

80 screening samples and 260 validation samples from children with medulloblastoma. All patients received standard therapy per German protocols.

Intervention

Comparative genomic hybridization microarray was performed on screening samples to identify chromosomal loci of interest. Fluorescence in situ hybridization was used for validation samples looking for these loci: chromosome 6q (loss and gain), 17q (gain and isochromosome i[17q]), and MYC/MYCN amplification.

Outcomes

Primary outcome was the prognostic significance of these genetic variations on OS and PFS. Secondary outcomes were classification of cytogenetic risk groups and hazard ratios for each group.

KEY RESULTS

- Hazard ratios for OS of cytogenetic risk groups were calculated with 6q and 17q balanced as a reference, (hazard ratio: 1.0) as follows:
  - 6q loss: 0.52 (95% CI 0.28–0.98)
  - 6q gain: 5.02 (95% CI 2.54–9.89)
  - MYC/MYCN amplification: 2.75 (95% CI 1.52–4.97)
- Incorporating molecular risk based on 17q/6q gain or MYC/MYCN amplification revealed significant variation in OS in the validation group ($p = 0.05$) and identified a large proportion of patients (72/234, 31%) with worse prognosis despite low clinical risk (arrow in curve shown in Fig. 42.1).

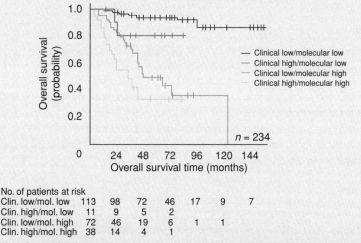

Figure 42.1 Simplified model of overall survival combining clinical (low vs. high) and molecular (low vs. high) risk. (From Pfister S, Remke M, Benner A, et al. Outcome prediction in pediatric medulloblastoma based on DNA copy-number aberrations of chromosomes 6q and 17q and the MYC and MYCN loci. *J Clin Oncol.* 2009;27(10):1627–1636, Figure 3.)

STUDY CONCLUSIONS

Identification of molecular markers in children with medulloblastoma allowed clinicians to more accurately identify those at high risk for disease progression and recurrence. In particular, 6q loss was associated with excellent prognosis while 6q gain, 17q gain, i(17q), and MYC/MYCN amplification portended a much worse prognosis than previously predicted.

COMMENTARY

This study provided a framework for incorporating molecular markers into risk stratification for pediatric medulloblastoma, adding significant prognostic value over traditional clinical staging alone. Current trials for pediatric medulloblastoma are seeking to further characterize loci of interest. In fact, a current trial is assigning risk grouping to patients at diagnosis by both clinical staging and molecular markers, including the absence of MYC/MYCN amplification.[1] Furthermore, a second trial is seeking to forego radiation therapy in low-risk patients, as determined by clinical and molecular criteria, the latter of which includes the absence of MYC/MYCN amplification and the presence of monosomy 6.[2]

Question

Do genetic aberrations alter prognosis of pediatric medulloblastoma?

Answer

When combined with currently used clinical staging factors, molecular markers greatly enhance prognostication in pediatric medulloblastoma, beginning to identify patients who require more robust initial therapy, as well as patients with low risk of disease recurrence for whom less aggressive therapy would mitigate morbidity without compromising remission rates.

References

1. Universitätsklinikum Hamburg-Eppendorf; Deutsche Kinderkrebsstiftung. *An International Prospective Study on Clinically Standard-risk Medulloblastoma in Children Older Than 3 to 5 Years With Low-risk Biological Profile (PNET 5 MB-LR) or Average-risk Biological Profile (PNET 5 MB-SR).* In: ClinicalTrials.gov [Internet]. Bethesda, MD: National Library of Medicine (US); 2000 (cited 2015 July 15). Available from: https://clinicaltrials.gov/ct2/show/NCT02066220. NLM Identifier: NCT02066220.
2. Sidney Kimmel Comprehensive Cancer Center; Johns Hopkins University. Pilot Study Assessing the Feasibility of a Surgery and Chemotherapy-Only Approach in the Upfront Therapy of Children With Wnt Positive Standard-Risk Medulloblastoma. In: ClinicalTrials.gov [Internet]. Bethesda, MD: National Library of Medicine (US). 2000 (cited 2015 July 15). Available from: https://clinicaltrials.gov/ct2/show/NCT02212574. NLM Identifier: NCT02212574.

PROPHYLACTIC TREATMENT WITH FACTOR VIII IN HEMOPHILIA

CHAPTER 43

Patricia A. Stoeck ■ Howard J. Weinstein

Prophylaxis Versus Episodic Treatment to Prevent Joint Disease in Boys With Severe Hemophilia

Manco-Johnson MJ, Abshire TC, Shapiro AD, et al. *N Engl J Med.* 2007;357(6):535–544

BACKGROUND

Hemophilia A, which can cause life-threatening bleeding, affects over 300,000 people worldwide. Hemarthrosis is the most common bleeding complication, comprising 70% to 80% of bleeding episodes.[1] With the development of recombinant products mitigating infection risk, some providers began using factor VIII (FVIII) prophylactically to prevent hemophilic arthropathy, rather than only during bleeding complications, as prevention has tremendous potential to improve quality of life and life expectancy. The timing, dosing, and duration of preventive therapy, however, were based on empiric guidelines, rather than objective studies, and cost remained a barrier.

OBJECTIVES

To determine if prophylactic FVIII infusions were superior to episodic FVIII for joint hemorrhage in preventing joint damage in boys with severe hemophilia A.

METHODS

Single-blind, randomized, multicenter trial from 1996 to 2005.

Patients

65 males ages <30 months with severe hemophilia A (FVIII level ≤2 U/dL). Select exclusion criteria: >2 joint hemorrhages into each index joint (ankle, knee, and elbow), abnormal joints on examination or imaging, presence of FVIII inhibitor, abnormal platelet counts.

Intervention

Prophylactic FVIII infusions (25 IU/kg every other day, 40 IU/kg when hemarthroses occurred) vs. episodic FVIII therapy (40 IU/kg when hemarthroses occurred, followed by 20 IU/kg at 24 and 72 hours, with the option of 20 IU/kg every other day for up to 4 weeks). Practitioners, radiologists, and laboratory technicians were blinded to treatment assignment and bleeding history.

Outcomes

Primary outcome was bone or cartilage damage in index joints on MRI or x-ray. Secondary outcomes included number of joint hemorrhages, extra-articular hemorrhages, and quantity of FVIII infusions.

KEY RESULTS

- 93% of the prophylaxis group vs. 55% of the episodic therapy group had normal index joints on MRI at age 6 ($p = 0.002$).
- Episodic therapy group had an RR of 6.1 (95% CI 1.5–24.4) of MRI-detected joint damage.
- Patients receiving prophylaxis had lower median number of annual joint hemorrhages (0.2 vs. 4.35) and total hemorrhages (1.15 vs. 17.13) as compared to episodic therapy ($p < 0.001$).

STUDY CONCLUSIONS

When started before age 30 months and continued until age 6, prophylactic infusions of recombinant FVIII were more effective than episodic therapy at preventing MRI-detectable hemophilic arthropathy.

COMMENTARY

This study demonstrated that prophylactic FVIII infusions had a major impact in reducing hemorrhages and permanent joint damage. Interestingly, the number of episodes of hemarthroses and joint examination scores did not correlate with MRI-detectable joint degeneration, suggesting that a partial benefit of prophylactic FVIII administration may be the prevention of ongoing, subclinical episodes of hemorrhage not previously recognized as contributing to joint damage. Furthermore, frequent hemarthroses prior to initiating prophylaxis may predispose patients to microhemorrhage or other mechanisms of injury that accelerate joint damage, which subsequent FVIII prophylaxis may not ameliorate.[2] These findings argue for initiating prophylaxis at an early age, prior to joint hemorrhage onset, a tenet now reflected in the World Federation of Hemophilia management guidelines.[1]

Question

Can prophylactic infusions of FVIII for boys with severe hemophilia A prevent future joint damage?

Answer

Yes. Children who received treatment only at the time of joint hemorrhage were 6 times more likely to have structural joint damage detected on MRI, as well as more likely to experience hemarthroses and extra-articular hemorrhages, compared to those receiving every other day prophylactic infusions beginning <30 months until age 6.

References

1. Srivastava A, Brewer AK, Mauser-Bunschoten EP, et al. Guidelines for the management of hemophilia. *Haemophilia.* 2013;19(1):e1–e47.
2. Roosendaal G, Lafeber F. Prophylactic treatment for prevention of joint disease in hemophilia—cost versus benefit. *N Engl J Med.* 2007;357(6):603–605.

SIGNIFICANCE OF MINIMAL RESIDUAL DISEASE IN ACUTE LYMPHOBLASTIC LEUKEMIA

Patricia A. Stoeck ■ Howard J. Weinstein

Clinical Significance of Minimal Residual Disease in Childhood Acute Lymphoblastic Leukemia and Its Relationship to Other Prognostic Factors: A Children's Oncology Group (COG) Study

Borowitz MJ, Devidas M, Hunger SP, et al. *Blood.* 2008;111(12):5477–5485

BACKGROUND

Minimal residual disease (MRD) has the potential to quickly identify acute lymphoblastic leukemia (ALL) patients at high risk for disease relapse and inform post-induction treatment strategies. Its role in predicting patient prognosis has been known since the mid-1990s, but it was not routinely incorporated into trial designs before 1999. Until this study, relative significance of MRD was unknown in comparison to other well-established factors for risk stratification, including age, white blood cell count (WBC) at diagnosis, genetic alterations, and post-induction bone marrow morphology.

OBJECTIVES

To assess the role of end-induction MRD in prognosis of childhood ALL, particularly in relation to previously demonstrated clinical and genetic features used for risk stratification.

METHODS

Prospective, multi-institutional study from 2000 to 2005.

Patients

1,971 children ages 1 to 21 years with precursor B-cell ALL (B-ALL). Select exclusion criteria: hypodiploidy, Philadelphia chromosome positive ALL, and induction failure.

Intervention

MRD on day 8 peripheral blood (PB-MRD) and day 29 bone marrow (BM-MRD) were measured by flow cytometry. MRD negativity was defined as ≤0.01% remaining leukemic cells. Known cytogenetic markers, including TEL-AML1 and trisomies 4 and 10 (double trisomies, DT), were evaluated. Analysis was then performed in combination with National Cancer Institute (NCI) risk grouping based on age, WBC at diagnosis, central nervous system disease, and testicular involvement to determine the prognostic ability of MRD in terms of event-free survival (EFS), early relapse (<3 years), and late relapse (≥3 years). No alterations in treatment schema were made due to PB- or BM-MRD.

Outcomes

Primary outcome was the prognostic significance of MRD on EFS and relapse. Secondary outcomes were interaction between day 8 PB-MRD and day 29 BM-MRD with other prognostic variables, including NCI risk group, TEL-AML1 translocation, and DT.

KEY RESULTS

- Day 29 BM-MRD positivity was a reliable predictor of relapses, both early (28% in MRD+ vs. 6.8% in MRD–; $p < 0.001$) and late (24% in MRD+ vs. 4.6% in MRD–; $p < 0.001$).
- Day 29 BM-MRD >0.01% was the most significant prognostic indicator (hazard ratio [HR] 4.31; $p < 0.001$).
- Patients with 0.01% to 0.1% day 29 MRD had worse outcomes compared with patients negative for MRD (59% ± 5% vs. 88% ± 1% 5-year EFS; $p < 0.001$).
- Other significant prognostic indicators included NCI risk group (HR 2.25; $p < 0.001$), DT (HR 0.57; $p < 0.001$), and day 8 PB-MRD >0.01% (HR 1.51; $p = 0.018$).

STUDY CONCLUSIONS

Day 29 BM-MRD was the single most influential prognostic variable in predicting EFS, early relapse, and late relapse in pediatric ALL.

COMMENTARY

While the potential value of MRD in anticipating outcomes for pediatric B-ALL was previously suspected, this was the first large study to specifically examine the magnitude of MRD's impact on prognosis, finding that it was even more predictive than NCI risk grouping or cytogenetics. Despite the changes in practice this study heralded, it remains important to place MRD in the context of other risk factors, as 51% of relapses occurred in day 29 BM-MRD negative patients. Nevertheless, this unique ability to obtain prognostic data in the first month of treatment has led to the consistent incorporation of both day 8 (PB) and day 29 (BM) MRD into risk stratification for childhood ALL.

Question

Is MRD positivity a significant prognostic indicator for pediatric patients with ALL?

Answer

Yes, day 29 bone marrow–MRD is the most significant prognostic factor in pediatric ALL. It has now been incorporated into risk stratification to guide subsequent treatment regimens.

INCREASED INCIDENCE OF CHRONIC DISEASE IN SURVIVORS OF CHILDHOOD CANCER

CHAPTER 45

Patricia A. Stoeck ■ Howard J. Weinstein

Chronic Health Conditions in Adult Survivors of Childhood Cancer

Oeffinger KC, Mertens AC, Sklar CA, et al. *N Eng J Med.* 2006;355(15):1572–1582

BACKGROUND
Through treatment improvements, the number of adult survivors of childhood cancer continues to grow, with an estimated 420,000 survivors in the United States currently.[1] However, these increased cure rates are not without morbidity. Previous studies identified some adverse health outcomes in cancer survivors, but had small sample sizes. This study used the Childhood Cancer Survivor Study (CCSS) to survey thousands of survivors for over 3 decades and collect data on several health conditions.

OBJECTIVES
To establish frequency and severity of chronic medical conditions in patients ≥5 years after treatment for childhood cancer and identify those at the highest risk for developing serious and incapacitating health conditions.

METHODS
Retrospective cohort study using CCSS data of patients diagnosed at 26 US centers between 1970 and 1986.

Patients
10,397 adult survivors of childhood malignancies (leukemia, central nervous system [CNS] tumor, Hodgkin disease, non-Hodgkin lymphoma, Wilms tumor, neuroblastoma, soft tissue sarcoma, and bone tumor). 3,034 nearest-age living siblings ≥18 years of age with no history of cancer served as controls. Select exclusion criteria: >21 years of age at diagnosis, <18 years of age at enrollment, and <5-year survival from diagnosis.

Intervention
137 health conditions were surveyed in both survivors and siblings. The severity of each condition was graded in severity from 1 (mild) to 5 (fatal). Medical records were reviewed.

Outcomes
Primary outcomes included the prevalence of any chronic medical condition, a severe or life-threatening condition (grade 3/4), and multiple health conditions. Secondary outcomes included relative risks of 10 specific conditions and risk of developing chronic conditions based on cancer type, exposure to a given therapeutic agent, and specific combinations of agents (including chemotherapy and radiation).

KEY RESULTS
- 62.3% of survivors had ≥1 chronic health conditions compared to 36.8% of siblings (RR 3.3, 95% CI 3.0–3.5).
- 27.5% of survivors vs. 5.2% of siblings had a severe or life-threatening condition (RR 8.2, 95% CI 6.9–9.7).
- Survivors of bone cancer (RR 38.9, 95% CI 31.2–48.5), CNS tumors (RR 12.6, 95% CI 10.3–15.5), and Hodgkin disease (RR 10.2, 95% CI 8.3–12.5) were much more likely to have severe or life-threatening conditions as compared to controls.

STUDY CONCLUSIONS
Adult survivors of childhood cancer had increased rates of chronic conditions and therefore require long-term health monitoring.

COMMENTARY

As more children with cancer are surviving to adulthood, the negative health outcomes secondary to chemotherapy and radiation therapy have become apparent. Despite its reliance on self-report and an incomplete list of chronic conditions (including the omission of mental health diagnoses), this study represents one of the first efforts for long-term monitoring of survivors of childhood cancer and highlighted the need to develop systems equipped to care for the specialized health needs of this population. These data from the CCSS, in conjunction with other studies, have led to the development of provider guidelines for care of survivors of childhood cancer.[1]

Question
How does the health status of adults with a previous history of childhood malignancy compare to those of age-matched controls?

Answer
Adult survivors of pediatric cancer are 3 times more likely than their unaffected siblings to have a chronic medical condition and are much more likely to have a debilitating or life-threatening ailment, thereby highlighting the importance of continued follow-up and monitoring for these complications.

Reference
1. Children's Oncology Group. *Long Term Follow Up Guidelines for Survivors of Childhood, Adolescence, and Young Adult Cancers, Version 4.0.* Monrovia, CA: Children's Oncology Group; 2013. Available on-line: www.survivorshipguidelines.org.

CHAPTER 46

TREATMENT OF ACUTE IDIOPATHIC THROMBOCYTOPENIC PURPURA

Patricia A. Stoeck ■ Howard J. Weinstein

Corticosteroids Versus Intravenous Immune Globulin for the Treatment of Acute Immune Thrombocytopenic Purpura in Children: A Systematic Review and Meta-Analysis of Randomized Controlled Trials

Beck CE, Nathan PC, Parkin PC, et al. *J Pediatr.* 2005;147(4):521–527

BACKGROUND

Although it is typically a self-limited condition, treatments for childhood immune thrombocytopenic purpura (ITP) have been pursued given the 0.2% to 1% risk of severe bleeding such as intracranial hemorrhage (ICH) with platelet counts $<20,000/mm^3$. Previous guidelines for ITP management in children were based on expert opinion and qualitative studies and included therapies such as IV immune globulin (IVIG), Rho(D) immune globulin corticosteroids, and supportive care alone. This study represents the first systematic review comparing IVIG to corticosteroids.

OBJECTIVES

To compare efficacy of IVIG versus corticosteroids in treatment of acute ITP.

METHODS

Systematic review and meta-analysis of 10 randomized controlled trials from 1985 to 2003.

Patients

615 patients ages 3 months to 18 years at the initial presentation of primary acute ITP. Select exclusion criteria: studies involving children with other causes of thrombocytopenia and prior ITP treatment.

Intervention

Administration of IVIG (0.4 to 1 g/kg/d for 1 to 5 days) vs. corticosteroids (methylprednisolone IV 10 to 30 mg/kg/d over 2 to 7 days or prednisone PO 2 to 4 mg/kg/d over 21 days, including taper). Platelet count following treatment initiation was measured.

Outcomes

Primary outcome was the number of patients with platelet counts $>20,000/mm^3$ 48 hours after treatment onset. Secondary outcomes were number of patients with platelet counts $>20,000/mm^3$ at 24 and 72 hours, development of chronic ITP, rates of ICH, mortality, and side effects.

KEY RESULTS

- At 48 hours, those treated with corticosteroids had a platelet count $\geq 20,000/mm^3$ less often than those treated with IVIG (RR 0.74, 95% CI 0.65–0.85).
- Number needed to treat (NNT) with IVIG to prevent one patient from having a platelet count $<20,000/mm^3$ at 48 hours was 4.55 (95% CI 3.23–7.69).
- RR of developing chronic ITP after corticosteroid therapy as compared to IVIG was 1.40 (95% CI 1.01–1.93).

STUDY CONCLUSIONS

IVIG was significantly more likely than corticosteroids to raise the platelet count $>20,000/mm^3$ 48 hours after acute ITP onset, making the risk of significant hemorrhage less likely.

COMMENTARY

This study represented the first effort to aggregate results of prior trials and suggested an advantage to therapy with IVIG for acute ITP. Determining a standard of care for managing severe thrombocytopenia is essential because lower platelet counts 48 hours after presentation are associated with higher risk of uncommon but serious adverse events such as major hemorrhage.[1] These study findings were incorporated into the guidelines from the American Society of Hematology in 2011, recommending IVIG over corticosteroids in cases where treatment is warranted.[2] Given the infrequency with which children develop clinically significant bleeding secondary to acute ITP, the impetus to treat based on platelet count alone or in the absence of clinically significant hemorrhage remains uncertain. Still, clinicians continue to favor treatment when there is mucocutaneous bleeding or platelet count $<10,000/mm^3$.

Question

In acute immune ITP, is IVIG or corticosteroids more likely to raise the platelet count $>20,000/mm^3$ 48 hours after starting treatment?

Answer

A patient is 26% more likely to reach a platelet count $>20,000/mm^3$ with IVIG, regardless of the dose of corticosteroid used. IVIG may decrease the risk of developing major hemorrhage or chronic ITP.

References

1. Medeiros D, Buchanan GR. Major hemorrhage in children with idiopathic thrombocytopenic purpura: Immediate response to therapy and long-term outcome. *J Pediatr.* 1998;133(3):334–339.
2. Neunert C, Lim W, Crowther M, et al. The American Society of Hematology 2011 evidence-based practice guideline for immune thrombocytopenia. *Blood.* 2011;117(16):4190–4207.

CHAPTER 47

HYDROXYUREA THERAPY IN SICKLE CELL ANEMIA

Juliana Mariani ■ Howard J. Weinstein

Long-Term Hydroxyurea Therapy for Infants With Sickle Cell Anemia: The HUSOFT Extension Study

Hankins JS, Ware RE, Rogers ZR, et al. *Blood.* 2005;106(7):2269–2275

BACKGROUND

Beginning as early as age 2, children with sickle cell anemia (SCA) can suffer from significant end-organ dysfunction related to their disease. Hydroxyurea is an antimetabolite agent that is known to increase levels of fetal hemoglobin (HbF) in pediatric and adult patients. The HUSOFT study was the first to show the feasibility and safety of hydroxyurea in infants with SCA after 2 years of treatment.[1] At the completion of that trial, however, little remained known about the long-term effects of higher doses of hydroxyurea or its possible efficacy in reducing irreversible end-organ dysfunction related to SCA, leading to this extension study.

OBJECTIVES

To assess the safety and efficacy of long-term hydroxyurea with dose escalation in young children with SCA.

METHODS

Prospective, multicenter, open-label, single-arm study at 5 US centers from 1996 to 1997.

Patients

21 patients ages 2 to 4 years with diagnosis of homozygous SCA (HbSS) or sickle β0-thalassemia who were previously enrolled in the HUSOFT pilot study. Select exclusion criteria: none.

Intervention

Treatment with hydroxyurea starting at 20 mg/kg/d with a dose escalation of 5 mg/kg every 6 months to a maximum dose of 30 mg/kg/d. Patients were monitored with routine physical examinations and laboratory testing and followed for up to 6 years of therapy.

Outcomes

Primary outcomes were hematologic efficacy and toxicity as compared to historical controls from the Cooperative Study of Sickle Cell Disease. Secondary outcomes were end-organ dysfunction (splenic sequestration, stroke, acute chest syndrome [ACS], and pain crises) and growth.

KEY RESULTS
- Percentage of HbF was higher after 4 years of hydroxyurea treatment vs. 2 years of treatment ($p < 0.05$).
- Hydroxyurea was tolerated in 95% of patients.
- HUSOFT patients had significantly decreased ACS incidence compared to historical controls (7.5 events/100 person-years vs. 24.5 events/100 person-years, $p = 0.001$).
- Only 43% (6/14) of patients who had baseline splenic function assessed had functional asplenia at study completion vs. 94% incidence of asplenia in age-matched untreated controls ($p < 0.001$).
- Boys had gains in growth during hydroxyurea treatment: they were at the 25th percentile for weight and 40th percentile for height at the start of therapy and reached the 50th percentile for both after 4 years of therapy.

STUDY CONCLUSIONS
Hydroxyurea at 30 mg/kg/d for up to 6 years was safe, increased HbF levels, and decreased ACS incidence in young children with SCA.

COMMENTARY
The original HUSOFT study demonstrated that the administration of hydroxyurea was feasible, nontoxic, and had quantifiable hematologic effects. HUSOFT extension showed sustained hematologic effects as well as a decrease in ACS and functional asplenia over a longer time period. For infants with SCA, hydroxyurea is now used in children with ≥3 admissions in a 12-month period, history of exchange transfusion, or history of ACS. Additionally, based on the results of the BABY HUG trial, hydroxyurea is recommended to begin as early as 9 months of age in symptomatic infants.[2]

Question
Is long-term use of hydroxyurea safe and beneficial for young children with SCA?

Answer
Hydroxyurea at 30 mg/kg/d is safe in infants with SCA and may help to prevent ACS and functional asplenia.

References
1. Wang WC, Wynn LW, Rogers ZR, et al. A two-year pilot trial of hydroxyurea in very young children with sickle-cell anemia. *J Pediatr.* 2001;139(6):790–796.
2. Wang WC, Ware RE, Miller ST, et al. Hydroxycarbamide in very young children with sickle-cell anaemia: A multicentre, randomised, controlled trial (BABY HUG). *Lancet.* 2011;377(9778):1663–1672.

SYMPTOM MANAGEMENT AT THE END OF LIFE IN PEDIATRIC ONCOLOGY

CHAPTER 48

Juliana Mariani ■ Howard J. Weinstein

Symptoms and Suffering at the End of Life in Children With Cancer

Wolfe J, Grier HE, Klar N, et al. *N Engl J Med.* 2000;342(5):326–333

BACKGROUND
There are 15,000 new pediatric cancer diagnoses and approximately 3,000 deaths annually making cancer the leading cause of nonaccidental death in childhood. Pediatric oncology patients often receive aggressive treatment with a goal of cure even at the end of life, raising concerns about whether care adequately addresses suffering. Palliative care services are part of the standard of care, though implementation varies. This study was one of the first to assess the practices and quality of end of life care in pediatric oncology.

OBJECTIVES
To describe the delivery of care and symptom presence and management in the last month of life, as well as factors related to suffering in pediatric patients with cancer.

METHODS
Interview of parents from 1997 to 1998 whose children died from cancer between 1990 and 1997 at 2 US academic centers.

Patients
107 parents whose children died >1 year prior. Select exclusion criteria: non-English speaking, living outside of North America.

Intervention
Data obtained from medical charts and structured parental interviews about the presence and severity of children's symptoms, including pain, poor appetite, nausea, vomiting, constipation, diarrhea, dyspnea, fatigue, and quality of life, as well as how these symptoms were managed. Parents were queried about physician involvement at end of life.

Outcomes
Primary outcomes were symptoms of suffering and quality of life measures related to mood, anxiety, and fear. Secondary outcome was physician involvement.

KEY RESULTS
- Two-thirds of children who died of progressive disease had a discussion of end of life care an average of 58.1 days before death.
- 49% of children died in the hospital and 45% of these children died in the ICU.
- 89% of parents reported that their child suffered "a lot" or a "great deal" from ≥1 symptom at the end of life and 51% from ≥3 symptoms.

- Parents were more likely than physicians to report that patients had fatigue, poor appetite, and constipation ($p < 0.001$).
- Lack of primary oncologist involvement was associated with significantly more suffering from pain (OR 2.6, 95% CI 1.0–6.7).

STUDY CONCLUSIONS

Children who died from cancer had significant suffering in the last month of life without adequate treatment of their symptoms.

COMMENTARY

This study underscores the importance of concurrently treating a child's disease, managing associated symptoms, and discussing end of life needs in pediatric oncology. Notable was the discrepancy in parent- versus physician-reported symptoms, suggesting that clinicians may not be as attuned to symptoms at the end of life as was previously believed. Shortly after the study's publication, the American Academy of Pediatrics published guidelines calling for palliative care programs to address needs of children with life-threatening or terminal conditions.[1] In the 10 years since the emergence of formal pediatric palliative care programs, there are now over 100. However, a recent study showed that only 58% of Children's Oncology Group member hospitals had such programs available, suggesting there is still room for improvement.[2]

Question

Is the care of children with cancer optimized at the end of life?

Answer

Not necessarily. The majority of pediatric cancer patients have significant suffering and symptoms which warrant close attention by the primary oncologist and support from palliative care and pain specialists.

References

1. American Academy of Pediatrics. Committee on Bioethics and Committee on Hospital Care. Palliative care for children. *Pediatrics.* 2000;106(2 Pt 1):351–357.
2. Johnston DL, Nagel K, Friedman DL, et al. Availability and use of palliative care and end-of-life services for pediatric oncology patients. *J Clin Oncol.* 2008;26(28):4646–4650.

CHAPTER 49

STROKE RISK REDUCTION IN SICKLE CELL ANEMIA

Juliana Mariani ■ Howard J. Weinstein

Prevention of a First Stroke by Transfusions in Children With Sickle Cell Anemia and Abnormal Results on Transcranial Doppler Ultrasonography

Adams RJ, Mckie VC, Hsu L, et al. *N Engl J Med.* 1998;339(1):5–11

BACKGROUND

Stroke occurs in 11% of patients with sickle cell anemia (SCA) by age 20.[1] Children at high risk for stroke have been identified using transcranial Doppler ultrasonography (TCD) screening. Although the use of blood transfusions to prevent recurrent stroke in SCA was established, the role in prevention of first stroke had not been investigated until this study.

OBJECTIVES

To assess the impact of blood transfusions on prevention of first stroke in children with SCA.

METHODS

Randomized controlled study at 14 US centers from 1995 to 1996.

Patients

130 children ages 2 to 16 years with SCA or sickle β0-thalassemia with abnormal TCD results (mean blood flow velocity of internal carotid or middle cerebral artery >200 cm/s on 2 ultrasounds). Select exclusion criteria: prior stroke, contraindication to chronic transfusion, conditions or treatments that increase stroke risk, ferritin >500 ng/mL.

Intervention

Standard care vs. administration of blood transfusions to reach a target of sickle hemoglobin (HbS) <30% within 21 days (without exceeding a hematocrit of 36%) via simple or exchange transfusions every 3 to 4 weeks. All patients received usual care including intermittent transfusions, but could not receive hydroxyurea or anti-sickling agents.

Outcomes

Primary outcome was incidence of neurologic events, specifically cerebral infarction and intracranial hemorrhage.

KEY RESULTS

- There were 10 cerebral infarctions and 1 cerebral hematoma out of 67 patients in the standard care group compared to 1 infarction in 63 patients in the transfusion group.

- Risk of stroke in the transfusion group was 92% lower as compared to standard care ($p < 0.001$).
- Rate of stroke in standard care group was 10% per year leading to early termination of the study.
- Mean serum ferritin levels in transfusion group increased from baseline of 164 + 155 ng/mL to 1,804 + 773 ng/mL at 12 months and 2,509 + 974 ng/mL at 24 months.
- There were 16 mild reactions to blood products and procedures. No transmission of hepatitis C, human immunodeficiency virus, or human T-lymphotropic virus 1 was documented.

STUDY CONCLUSIONS

Blood transfusions greatly reduced the risk of first stroke in children with SCA or sickle β0-thalassemia with prior abnormal results on TCD.

COMMENTARY

This pivotal study was the first to identify that children with SCA and abnormal TCD results benefit from prophylactic blood transfusions to prevent first stroke. The results were so profound that the trial was stopped prematurely. However, concerns were raised regarding the indefinite duration of chronic transfusions and related adverse effects, specifically iron overload. This prompted the STOP2 trial which attempted to identify patients who could potentially discontinue transfusions after TCD normalization, but found that patients in whom transfusions were discontinued had a recurrent increased stroke risk.[2] Current studies are evaluating hydroxyurea as an alternative to chronic transfusions.

Question

Are transfusions beneficial at preventing first stroke in patients with SCA with abnormal TCD?

Answer

Yes. However, there are significant risks associated with transfusions and this decision should be made after a thoughtful discussion with patients, parents, and providers.

References

1. Ohene-Frempong K, Weiner SJ. Cerebrovascular accidents in sickle cell disease: Rates and risk factors. *Blood.* 1998;91(1):288–294.
2. Adams RJ, Brambilla D; Optimizing Primary Stroke Prevention in Sickle Cell Anemia (STOP 2) Trial Investigators. Discontinuing prophylactic transfusions used to prevent stroke in sickle cell disease. *N Engl J Med.* 2005;353(26):2769–2778.

INFECTIOUS DISEASES

50. Management of Community-Acquired Skin Abscesses

51. Sequential Therapy in the Treatment of Osteomyelitis

52. Impact of Antibiotic Pretreatment on Cerebrospinal Fluid Profiles

53. Concomitant Bacterial Infection in Infants With Respiratory Syncytial Virus

54. High-Dose Acyclovir for Neonatal Herpes Simplex Virus Infection

55. Clinical Prediction Algorithm for Septic Arthritis

56. Oral Versus Intravenous Therapy for Urinary Tract Infections

57. Palivizumab for Reduction of Respiratory Syncytial Virus Infections

58. Reduction in Mother-to-Child Transmission of Human Immunodeficiency Virus

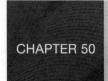

MANAGEMENT OF COMMUNITY-ACQUIRED SKIN ABSCESSES

CHAPTER 50

Rebecca Cook ■ Chadi M. El Saleeby

Randomized, Controlled Trial of Antibiotics in the Management of Community-Acquired Skin Abscesses in the Pediatric Patient

Duong M, Markwell S, Peter J, et al. *Ann Emerg Med.* 2010;55(5):401–407

BACKGROUND

The incidence of pediatric skin and soft tissue infections (SSTI) has tripled in the last decade. This is due in part to the prevalence of methicillin-resistant *Staphylococcus aureus* (MRSA), which accounted for nearly 60% of *S. aureus* infections in children in 2007.[1] Incision and drainage (I&D) had been considered definitive treatment of skin abscesses, but with rising rates of community-acquired MRSA (CA-MRSA), there was concern that I&D alone was insufficient. This was the first randomized trial in children in the era of CA-MRSA that investigated whether antibiotics after I&D improved outcomes.

OBJECTIVES

To assess whether oral antibiotics after I&D of skin abscesses impact rates of treatment failure and recurrent infection.

METHODS

Double-blind, randomized, placebo-controlled noninferiority trial in a single pediatric emergency department (ED) from 2006 to 2008.

Patients

149 patients ages 3 months to 18 years with clinical or ultrasound diagnosis of skin abscess(es) undergoing I&D. Select exclusion criteria: toxic appearance, chronic medical illness, immunosuppression, recent antibiotics.

Intervention

After I&D, subjects were randomized to 10 days of trimethoprim-sulfamethoxazole (TMP-SMX; 10–12 mg/kg/d TMP divided twice daily, max 160 mg/dose) or placebo. Wound cultures were obtained and patients received standard wound care instructions. Follow-up consisted of phone calls at 2–3 days and 90 days, with medication adherence determined by bottle review at a 10- to 14-day visit.

Outcomes

Primary outcome was treatment failure at first follow-up (further surgical drainage, medication change, admission for IV antibiotics, new abscess located <5 cm from original abscess). Secondary outcomes were development of new infection, spread to household contacts, and adverse medication effects.

KEY RESULTS
- Placebo was noninferior to antibiotic with failure rates of 5.3% vs. 4.1%, respectively (difference of 1.2%, 1-sided CI $-\infty$ to 6.8).
- Antibiotic treatment yielded a lower incidence of new abscesses at 10-day follow-up (12.9% vs. 26.4%; difference of 13.5%, 1-sided CI $-\infty$ to 24.3); however, this difference did not persist at 90 days (28.3% vs. 28.8%; difference of 0.5%, 1-sided CI $-\infty$ to 15.6).
- Side effect rates were similar in both groups.
- 80% of the pathogens isolated were MRSA, all TMP-SMX susceptible.

STUDY CONCLUSIONS
Even with rising rates of CA-MRSA SSTIs, TMP-SMX treatment following I&D yielded similar failure rates as compared to placebo. While a lower proportion of children who received oral antibiotics developed new lesions at 10 to 14 days, this benefit was not observed in longer-term follow-up.

COMMENTARY
Although a single-center trial, these results argue against antibiotic use in patients with uncomplicated skin abscesses. This is particularly relevant given issues of medication adherence, rising antibiotic resistance, healthcare costs, and medication side effects. This study is limited by reliance on telephone follow-ups, and 35% loss to follow-up at 3 months. The generalizability is also limited by the preponderance of patients with abscess in the diaper area. Nonetheless, it demonstrates that abscess drainage may be sufficient to achieve cure. Of note, the high incidence of relapse in both groups highlights the need for better approaches to MRSA decolonization, an area of ongoing investigation.

Question
Is I&D alone equivalent to I&D followed by TMP-SMX for treatment of uncomplicated community-acquired skin abscesses?

Answer
Yes, I&D alone is not inferior to I&D plus oral antibiotics for the treatment of simple abscesses in otherwise healthy children.

Reference
1. Gerber JS, Coffin SE, Smathers SA, et al. Trends in the incidence of methicillin-resistant Staphylococcus aureus infection in children's hospitals in the United States. *Clin Infect Dis.* 2009;49(1):65–71.

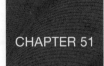

SEQUENTIAL THERAPY IN THE TREATMENT OF OSTEOMYELITIS

CHAPTER 51

Rebecca Cook ■ Chadi M. El Saleeby

Prolonged Intravenous Therapy Versus Early Transition to Oral Antimicrobial Therapy for Acute Osteomyelitis in Children
Zaoutis T, Localio AR, Leckerman K, et al. *Pediatrics.* 2009;123(2):636–642

BACKGROUND

Osteomyelitis accounts for up to 1% of pediatric hospitalizations in the US. Inadequate treatment leads to serious morbidity including chronic infection and permanent bone injury, with associated consequences for growth and function in children. Expert consensus had recommended 4 to 6 weeks of IV antibiotic treatment for acute osteomyelitis in children, which was costly and carried risks from long-term central venous catheters. Small case series and one systematic review suggested that sequential therapy, a short course of IV antibiotics followed by oral antibiotics, yielded equivalent outcomes to IV therapy alone, but this was the first study to directly compare these approaches.

OBJECTIVES

To compare treatment outcomes in children who receive sequential therapy vs. prolonged IV antibiotics for acute osteomyelitis.

METHODS

Retrospective, single-blinded cohort study in 29 US children's hospitals from 2000 to 2005.

Patients

1,969 children ages 2 months to 17 years hospitalized for acute or unspecified osteomyelitis. Select exclusion criteria: chronic osteomyelitis, comorbid conditions suggesting complicated osteomyelitis, length of hospitalization >10 days.

Intervention

Early transition from IV to oral antibiotics (sequential therapy) vs. prolonged IV therapy identified by billing code for central venous catheterization, with 10% of charts randomly sampled to confirm accuracy.

Outcomes

Primary outcome was treatment failure (rehospitalization within 6 months with codes for acute or chronic osteomyelitis, osteomyelitis complications, or musculoskeletal surgical procedure). Secondary outcomes included all rehospitalizations within 6 months, catheter-related complications, and adverse reactions to antibiotics.

KEY RESULTS
- Proportion of children transitioned to oral therapy varied significantly across hospitals from 10% to 95% ($p < 0.001$).
- Treatment failure rates were not significantly different between therapy groups: 5% (54/1,021) of children in prolonged IV therapy group compared to 4% (38/94) of children in the sequential therapy group.
- Children in the prolonged IV therapy group were more likely to experience a treatment-related complication, including rehospitalization for any cause (10% vs. 6%, $p = 0.017$), readmission for antimicrobial complications (1.6% vs. 0.4%, $p = 0.005$), or readmission for catheter-related complications (3%).

STUDY CONCLUSIONS
Sequential therapy for acute uncomplicated osteomyelitis was therapeutically equivalent to prolonged IV therapy and avoided the risks of secondary complications associated with IV antibiotics and central venous catheters.

COMMENTARY
Although retrospective, this was the first large study demonstrating that sequential therapy was as effective as prolonged IV therapy, leading to sequential antibiotic therapy becoming common practice in patients with acute uncomplicated osteomyelitis. Based on this study and expert opinion, children who have rapid responses in clinical and laboratory parameters are now typically transitioned to oral agents after 5 to 7 days of IV therapy. Study limitations included a high patient exclusion rate and a predominance of pelvic and lower extremity osteomyelitis. There was concern for selection bias as physicians may have chosen healthier patients to transition to oral antibiotics; however, the wide interhospital variability suggests that the use of sequential therapy was less patient specific and more based on local practices. High-quality evidence on the timing of transition, optimal antimicrobial choice, and total therapy duration is still lacking.

Question
Is early transition to oral antibiotics after initial IV therapy safe and effective in children with acute osteomyelitis?

Answer
Yes. Children with acute, uncomplicated osteomyelitis may be transitioned from IV to oral therapy after 5 to 7 days. With this approach, there are similar rates of treatment failure but a significantly decreased risk of secondary complications making this the preferred method for therapy.

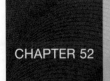

IMPACT OF ANTIBIOTIC PRETREATMENT ON CEREBROSPINAL FLUID PROFILES

CHAPTER 52

Rebecca Cook ■ Chadi M. El Saleeby

Effect of Antibiotic Pretreatment on Cerebrospinal Fluid Profiles of Children With Bacterial Meningitis

Nigrovic LE, Malley R, Macias CG, et al. *Pediatrics*. 2008;122(4):726–730

BACKGROUND

Treatment with antibiotics before sampling cerebrospinal fluid (CSF) complicates the interpretation of CSF parameters including cell counts, chemistries, and cultures in children with bacterial meningitis. Prior data on the impact of antibiotic pretreatment were published before vaccines against *Haemophilus influenzae* type b and *Streptococcus pneumoniae* became widely available. This study sought to reassess the impact of antibiotics on CSF parameters in the conjugate vaccine era.

OBJECTIVES

To evaluate the effect of antibiotic pretreatment on the CSF profiles of children with bacterial meningitis.

METHODS

Retrospective cohort study at 20 pediatric emergency departments (ED) from 2001 to 2004.

Patients

245 children ages 1 month to 18 years diagnosed with definite bacterial meningitis (positive CSF culture, or CSF pleocytosis ≥10 white blood cells [WBC]/μL with positive blood culture or CSF latex agglutination test) or probable bacterial meningitis (positive CSF Gram stain with negative blood or CSF cultures). Select exclusion criteria: CSF shunt, recent neurosurgery, or immunosuppression.

Intervention

Comparison of CSF parameters of the pretreatment group (oral or IV antibiotic therapy <72 hours before CSF sampling) and no antibiotic group.

Outcomes

Primary outcomes included change in CSF studies (WBC, absolute neutrophil count [ANC], protein, glucose, Gram stain, and culture) between groups and over time in relation to duration of pretreatment.

KEY RESULTS

- 231 children had definite and 14 had probable bacterial meningitis. Overall, 85/245 (35%) received antibiotic pretreatment.
- When pretreated patients were compared to those who did not receive antibiotics, the rates of positive CSF Gram stains were similar, but there was a lower frequency of positive CSF cultures (70% vs. 88%, $p = 0.001$).
- CSF WBC and ANC measurements were not significantly different between children who did and did not receive antibiotic pretreatment at any time point up to 72 hours.
- CSF chemistries normalized with pretreatment: glucose significantly increased ($p = 0.005$) and CSF protein significantly decreased ($p = 0.008$) for children who received antibiotic pretreatment ≥12 hours prior to CSF sampling.

STUDY CONCLUSIONS

In children pretreated with antibiotics, CSF Gram stain, WBC, and ANC remained diagnostically valuable as they did not significantly change within 72 hours of starting therapy. Antibiotic pretreatment was associated with a trend toward normalization of the CSF glucose and protein and increased rate of CSF culture sterility.

COMMENTARY

While this is a retrospective study, it sampled a large and geographically diverse population with rigorous criteria for defining bacterial meningitis. It demonstrated that CSF pleocytosis persisted in children with bacterial meningitis after pretreatment, but that protein and glucose measurements changed within 12 hours of antibiotic therapy, making CSF chemistries unreliable for diagnosis in this population. Of note, this study was not sufficiently powered to detect differences in relation to specific antibiotics given or routes of administration. Overall, CSF sampling yields useful information if performed within 72 hours of starting antibiotic therapy and preferably within 12 hours in order to utilize glucose and protein in assessment for meningitis.

Question

Is CSF sampling with lumbar puncture after administration of antibiotics still of diagnostic utility?

Answer

Yes. Although ideally sampling would be performed within 12 hours, and it does reduce the yield from bacterial cultures, pretreatment with oral or IV antibiotics within 72 hours of the lumbar puncture does not significantly affect the CSF WBC count, ANC, or Gram stain.

CONCOMITANT BACTERIAL INFECTION IN INFANTS WITH RESPIRATORY SYNCYTIAL VIRUS

CHAPTER 53

Juliana Mariani ■ Chadi M. El Saleeby

Risk of Serious Bacterial Infection in Young Febrile Infants With Respiratory Syncytial Virus Infections

Levine DA, Platt SL, Dayan PS, et al. *Pediatrics.* 2004;113(6):1728–1734

BACKGROUND

Febrile infants ≤60 days old are at high risk for serious bacterial infections (SBIs), including meningitis, bacteremia, and urinary tract infections (UTIs). It was unclear whether young infants with documented respiratory syncytial virus (RSV) infection also had a similarly elevated risk.

OBJECTIVES

To assess the risk of SBIs in febrile infants with RSV as compared to those without RSV.

METHODS

Prospective cross-sectional study in 8 US centers from 1998 to 2001.

Patients

1,248 febrile (≥38°C) infants ≤60 days old presenting to a pediatric emergency department. Select exclusion criteria: antibiotics ≤48 hours prior to presentation, no bacterial cultures or RSV testing obtained.

Intervention

Patients underwent history and physical examination, nasopharyngeal swab for RSV rapid antigen detection, complete blood count with differential and cultures of blood, urine, and cerebrospinal fluid (CSF).

Outcomes

Primary outcome was overall risk of SBI in infants with and without RSV infection. Secondary outcomes included rates of individual bacterial infections and rates of SBI by age category (≤28 days vs. 29 to 60 days) and by RSV status.

KEY RESULTS

- Of 1,248 patients, 269 (22%) were RSV positive. Lumbar punctures were performed in 1,164 (93%), blood cultures in 1,235 (99%), and urine cultures in 1,227 (98%).

- RSV-positive infants were less likely to have any SBI compared with RSV-negative infants (7% vs. 12.5%; RR 0.6, 95% CI 0.3–0.9). They also were less likely to have bacteremia than RSV-negative infants (1.1% vs. 2.3%, respectively). None had bacterial meningitis.
- RSV-positive infants did have an appreciable rate of UTI though less than that in RSV-negative infants (5.4% vs. 10.1%; risk difference 4.7%, 95% CI 1.4–8.1).
- In subgroup analysis of infants <1 month of age, the overall rate of SBI was unaffected by RSV status (10.1% in RSV-positive vs. 14.2% in RSV-negative, 95% CI 0.35–1.5).

STUDY CONCLUSIONS

Febrile RSV-positive infants ≤60 days of age remained at risk for SBIs, particularly UTIs, although risk was significantly lower than in RSV-negative infants.

COMMENTARY

This study shows RSV status to be an independent predictor for SBIs in infants, necessitating its inclusion in the evaluation pathway. However, in infants <1 month of age, the risk of SBI is unaffected, thus supporting the standard practice of a full infectious evaluation in all febrile neonates, irrespective of RSV status. In an otherwise well-appearing febrile RSV-positive infant between the age of 1 to 3 months with low-risk criteria for SBI, an LP may not be needed and blood and urine sampling may suffice. The results of this study were also validated in an outpatient setting.[1] Of note, the original study did not include bacterial pneumonia as an SBI, and did not test for other viral infections such as influenza, which may help to further categorize SBI risk factors in these age groups.

Question

How does the risk of SBIs in RSV-positive infants ≤60 days compare to infants without RSV?

Answer

In febrile neonates, the risk of SBI is unaffected by RSV status, necessitating a full sepsis evaluation and empiric antibiotics. However, in patients older than 1 month although UTIs remain a concern regardless of RSV status, there is a lower risk of all SBIs in RSV-positive infants compared to RSV-negative patients.

Reference

1. Luginbuhl LM, Newman TB, Pantell RH, et al. Office-based treatment and outcomes for febrile infants with clinically diagnosed bronchiolitis. *Pediatrics.* 2008;122(5):947–954.

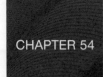

HIGH-DOSE ACYCLOVIR FOR NEONATAL HERPES SIMPLEX VIRUS INFECTION

CHAPTER 54

Juliana Mariani ■ Chadi M. El Saleeby

Safety and Efficacy of High-Dose Intravenous Acyclovir in the Management of Neonatal Herpes Simplex Virus Infections

Kimberlin DW, Lin CY, Jacobs RF, et al. *Pediatrics.* 2001;108(2):230–238

BACKGROUND
Neonatal herpes simplex virus (HSV) infection occurs in 1:3,000 to 1:20,000 live births, with 3 different phenotypes of illness: skin, eye, and mucous membranes (SEM), central nervous system (CNS) disease (meningoencephalitis), and disseminated disease affecting multiple organs. IV acyclovir (ACV) was approved by the Food and Drug Administration (FDA) in 1998 for neonatal HSV treatment; the initial dosing regimen, extrapolated from adult studies, was 30 mg/kg/d IV divided every 8 hours (standard dose, SD). Complications of HSV, however, remained unacceptably high: patients with disseminated disease had a mortality risk of ~40% at 1 year of life, and up to 50% of survivors of HSV meningoencephalitis had significant morbidity subsequently.

OBJECTIVES
To assess the safety and efficacy of higher doses of ACV in the treatment of neonatal HSV disease.

METHODS
Phase 2 open-label prospective multicenter trial in the US and Mexico from 1989 to 1997.

Patients
88 neonates ≤28 days old with weight ≥1,200 g and gestation >32 weeks. 69 had CNS or disseminated HSV; 19 additional patients had SEM or a clinical diagnosis and were included on a compassionate basis. Select exclusion criteria: receipt of other antiviral medications.

Intervention
IV ACV at intermediate dose (ID, 45 mg/kg/d) vs. high dose (HD, 60 mg/kg/d) divided 3 times daily for 21 days. Patients who had received 10 days of SD from a prior study by the investigators were reviewed for comparative analyses. Patients with culture- or PCR-confirmed HSV disease were included in efficacy analyses; all were included in safety analyses.

Outcomes
Primary outcomes were efficacy and safety of HD and ID ACV compared to historical controls who received SD ACV. Secondary outcomes were mortality and morbidity.

KEY RESULTS

- More patients with disseminated disease survived in the HD group than in the SD group (69% vs. 39%; OR 3.3, $p = 0.0035$). Patients in the ID and SD groups had statistically similar survival rates.
- After controlling for potential confounders, all patients treated with HD ACV were 6.6 times more likely to be developmentally normal at 12 months of age than patients on SD (95% CI 0.8–113.6).
- 21% (6/29) of infants who received HD ACV experienced neutropenia; all recovered during or after completion of treatment.

STUDY CONCLUSIONS

A 21-day course of HD ACV improved mortality and morbidity in infants with neonatal HSV infection without lasting adverse effects.

COMMENTARY

This landmark study led to revised dosing recommendations for infants with suspected HSV disease. However, the optimal length of therapy remains unclear, as patients in this study received treatment for 21 days, compared to 10 days for historical controls. The American Academy of Pediatrics Red Book now recommends HD ACV for 2 to 3 weeks for HSV infection between birth and 3 months of age.[1] Higher doses are now also routinely used for older individuals; the FDA has approved use of HD ACV for patients up to 12 years old with HSV meningoencephalitis. Bone marrow and kidney function should be carefully monitored for all age groups on HD ACV therapy.

Question

Is high-dose ACV efficacious and safe for the treatment of neonatal HSV infection?

Answer

IV ACV (60 mg/kg/d divided every 8 hours) for 2 to 3 weeks is the therapy of choice for all forms of neonatal HSV disease, with close monitoring of absolute neutrophil count in critically ill children.

Reference

1. American Academy of Pediatrics. Herpes simplex. In: Kimberlin DW, Brady MT, Jackson MA, Long SS, eds. *Red Book: 2015 Report of the Committee on Infectious Diseases.* 30th ed. Elk Grove, IL: American Academy of Pediatrics; 2015:432–445.

CHAPTER 55

CLINICAL PREDICTION ALGORITHM FOR SEPTIC ARTHRITIS

Matthew G. Gartland ■ Chadi M. El Saleeby

Differentiating Between Septic Arthritis and Transient Synovitis of the Hip in Children: An Evidence-Based Clinical Prediction Algorithm

Kocher MS, Zurakowski D, Kasser JR. *J Bone Joint Surg Am.* 1999;81(12):1662–1670

BACKGROUND

With delay in diagnosis, septic arthritis (SA) in children may be complicated by joint restriction, bone necrosis, and pathologic fractures. Early diagnosis, however, remains a challenge as there are many benign mimicking conditions. This study sought to establish a simple algorithm to distinguish between 2 common but therapeutically disparate pathologies: SA and transient synovitis (TS).

OBJECTIVES

To develop an evidence-based clinical algorithm to differentiate between SA and TS of the hip in ambulatory children.

METHODS

Retrospective cohort study in a single US center from 1979 to 1996.

Patients

168 children (mean age 5.6 years) with acute hip pain presenting to the emergency department. Select exclusion criteria: underlying immunocompromise, rheumatologic disease, adjacent osteomyelitis, fracture or other anatomical abnormalities on x-ray, or no CBC or adequate joint fluid evaluation performed.

Intervention

General demographic and clinical data were extracted from medical records: fever, recent infection and antibiotic use, weight-bearing status, erythrocyte sedimentation rate (ESR), serum white blood cell count (WBC), and radiographic findings.

Outcomes

Primary outcomes were true SA (positive joint fluid or blood culture, and joint fluid WBC ≥50,000 cells/mm^3), presumed SA (negative cultures but joint WBC ≥50,000 cells/mm^3), and TS (WBC <50,000 cells/mm^3, negative blood and joint fluid cultures, and resolution of symptoms).

KEY RESULTS

- On multivariable analyses, fever (oral temperature ≥38.5°C), non-weight-bearing status, ESR >40 mm/h, and WBC ≥12,000 cells/mm^3 all significantly predicted

SA. The area under the receiver-operating characteristic curve was 0.96 with inclusion of these variables, indicating excellent diagnostic performance for sensitivity and specificity.
- When all 4 criteria were present, the predicted probability of SA of the hip was 99.6%. The probability was 93.1%, 40.0%, 3.0%, and 0.2% in children with 3, 2, 1, and 0 predictors, respectively.

STUDY CONCLUSIONS
SA of the hip could be differentiated from TS using a constellation of simple clinical and laboratory criteria.

COMMENTARY

This study combined 4 simple variables (often referred to as "Kocher criteria") into a straightforward and effective clinical decision-making tool that was subsequently validated in a prospective analysis.[1] Of note, this tool does not apply to patients who are nonambulatory at baseline and has not been validated for other joints. Adding C-reactive protein (CRP) demonstrated a similar performance of these criteria, with a predictive probability of 95.7%.[2] To date, there remains no clinical prediction rule validated in larger, multicenter, prospective studies that unequivocally differentiates between SA and TS. However, given that relevant data can be easily and rapidly obtained, these criteria in addition to elevated CRP can guide rapid decision making in children with an acutely irritable hip and identify those who need additional diagnostics and timely therapeutics.

Question
Can SA be differentiated from TS in children with acute hip pain using readily available clinical and laboratory data?

Answer
A predictive score combining fever, non–weight-bearing status, elevated ESR and CRP, and elevated WBC can help differentiate SA and TS. An aggressive pursuit of further diagnostics should be made when 4 or more criteria are present or significant clinical concern exists.

References
1. Kocher MS, Mandiga R, Zurakowski D, et al. Validation of a clinical prediction rule for the differentiation between septic arthritis and transient synovitis of the hip in children. *J Bone Joint Surg Am.* 2004;86-A(8): 1629–1635.
2. Caird MS, Flynn JM, Leung YL, et al. Factors distinguishing septic arthritis from transient synovitis of the hip in children. A prospective study. *J Bone Joint Surg Am.* 2006;88(6):1251–1257.

ORAL VERSUS INTRAVENOUS THERAPY FOR URINARY TRACT INFECTIONS

Matthew G. Gartland ■ Chadi M. El Saleeby

Oral Versus Initial Intravenous Therapy for Urinary Tract Infections in Young Febrile Children

Hoberman A, Wald ER, Hickey RW, et al. *Pediatrics.* 1999;104(1):79–86

BACKGROUND

In young children, urinary tract infections (UTI) may cause serious complications, including permanent scarring and diminished kidney function. Historically, there has been significant heterogeneity both in management with IV vs. PO antibiotic treatment and in duration of therapy.

OBJECTIVES

To compare the efficacy of PO antibiotic therapy alone versus sequential IV to PO treatment in young children with febrile UTI.

METHODS

Nonblinded randomized trial at 4 US centers from 1992 to 1997.

Patients

309 children ages 1 to 24 months with fever $\geq 38.3°C$, pyuria, bacteriuria, and growth of $\geq 50,000$ colony forming units (CFU)/mL on culture from a catheterized sample. Select exclusion criteria: Gram-positive cocci in urine, alternative source of fever, underlying chronic disease, severe illness, history of UTI, or structural urinary tract abnormality.

Intervention

Patients received a 14-day course of cefixime 8 mg/kg/d PO (double-strength dose on day 1) vs. cefotaxime 200 mg/kg/d IV for 3 days (or until afebrile for ≥ 24 hours, whichever longer), followed by cefixime PO to complete 14 days. Both groups then received prophylaxis with cefixime (4 mg/kg once daily) for 2 weeks until completion of a voiding cystourethrogram (VCUG). Children with vesicoureteral reflux (VUR) of grade 2 or higher were maintained on prophylaxis for 11 months, or until the reflux was grade 1 or resolved.

Outcomes

Primary short-term outcomes were urine sterilization at 24 hours and time to defervescence. Primary long-term outcomes were infection recurrence, renal scarring, and scarring extent on 6-month ^{99m}Tc-dimercaptosuccinic acid scan. Therapy cost was evaluated in both groups.

KEY RESULTS

- All urine cultures at 24 hours were sterile in both groups and mean time to defervescence was similar (24.7 hours PO vs. 23.9 hours IV/PO, $p = 0.76$).
- Rates of reinfection (4.6% PO vs. 7.2% IV/PO, $p = 0.28$), and renal scarring (9.8% PO vs. 7.2% IV/PO, $p = 0.21$) were similar between the 2 groups.
- Bacteremia rates were low, with no significant difference between groups (3.4% PO vs. 5.3% IV/PO, $p = 0.62$).
- Total costs were lower for the PO group than the IV/PO group ($1,473 vs. $3,577).

STUDY CONCLUSIONS

PO therapy for febrile UTI in children ages 1 to 24 months was equally effective and less costly than sequential (IV/PO) therapy.

COMMENTARY

This study provided support for treating febrile UTI in children <2 years solely with an oral agent, signifying a major practice change. Subsequent data have confirmed these results.[1] In updated 2011 guidelines, the American Academy of Pediatrics (AAP) now recognizes the equivalency of oral and sequential therapies, and states that otherwise healthy infants older than 1 month may be treated safely as outpatients using oral therapy.[2] Additionally, the AAP recommends limited imaging: kidney ultrasonography for all patients, but VCUG only in the setting of an abnormal ultrasound or recurrent UTIs. However, there remains a paucity of data regarding optimal management in complex populations including neonates, those with bacteremia, and those with renal abscesses.

Question

Is treatment with PO antibiotics effective for febrile UTI in young children?

Answer

Yes. In children older than 1 month and without sepsis, long- and short-term outcomes were similar in a well-designed randomized controlled trial comparing exclusive PO to sequential IV/PO therapy.

References

1. Bocquet N, Sergent Alaoui A, Jais JP, et al. Randomized trial of oral versus sequential IV/oral antibiotic for acute pyelonephritis in children. *Pediatrics.* 2012;129(2):e269–e275.
2. Subcommittee on Urinary Tract Infection, Steering Committee on Quality Improvement and Management, Roberts KB. Urinary tract infection: Clinical practice guideline for the diagnosis and management of the initial UTI in febrile infants and children 2 to 24 months. *Pediatrics.* 2011;128(3):595–610.

| CHAPTER 57 | # PALIVIZUMAB FOR REDUCTION OF RESPIRATORY SYNCYTIAL VIRUS INFECTIONS |

Molly Miloslavsky ■ Chadi M. El Saleeby

Palivizumab, a Humanized Respiratory Syncytial Virus Monoclonal Antibody, Reduces Hospitalization From Respiratory Syncytial Virus Infection in High-Risk Infants. The IMpact-RSV Study Group

Pediatrics. 1998;102(3 Pt 1):531–537

BACKGROUND

In the US, respiratory syncytial virus (RSV) is the leading cause of respiratory illness in infants and children under age 2. Risk factors for severe disease include prematurity, chronic lung disease (CLD), and hemodynamically significant cardiac lesions. Prior to this study, RSV IV immunoglobulin (RSV-IVIG) was shown to be effective RSV prophylaxis in high-risk pediatric patients.[1] However, long infusion time precluded widespread use. Palivizumab, a humanized monoclonal antibody, was an attractive alternative as it had potent anti-RSV activity in vitro and could be given intramuscularly (IM).

OBJECTIVES

To determine the safety and efficacy of IM palivizumab as RSV prophylaxis in high-risk infants.

METHODS

Double-blind, randomized, placebo-controlled trial in 139 centers in the US, Canada, and the United Kingdom from 1996 to 1997.

Patients

1,502 children age ≤6 months with history of prematurity ≤35 weeks' gestation or age ≤24 months with a history of bronchopulmonary dysplasia (BPD) requiring supplemental oxygen, corticosteroids, bronchodilators, or diuretics in the past 6 months. Select exclusion criteria: significant congenital heart disease, recent or active RSV infection.

Intervention

Patients were randomized to receive IM injections of either palivizumab 15 mg/kg ($n = 1,002$) or placebo ($n = 500$) every 30 days for 5 months during local RSV season. Patients were followed until 30 days after the last injection.

Outcomes

Primary outcome was incidence of hospitalization with confirmed RSV infection. Secondary outcomes were duration of hospitalization, time on supplemental oxygen, time with moderate-to-severe lower respiratory tract illness, and need for intensive care/mechanical ventilation.

KEY RESULTS

- Monthly palivizumab prophylaxis as compared to placebo resulted in overall reduction in hospitalization due to RSV (4.8% vs. 10.6%, $p < 0.00004$). Reductions were also seen in infants with prematurity (1.8% vs. 8.1%, $p < 0.001$) and BPD (7.9% vs. 12.8%, $p = 0.038$).
- Per 100 patients, infants receiving palivizumab had fewer total hospital days (36.4 vs. 62.6, $p < 0.001$), days on supplemental oxygen (30.3 vs. 50.6, $p < 0.001$), and days with a Lower Respiratory Tract Illness score ≥ 3 (29.6 vs. 47.4, $p < 0.001$).
- There were no differences in adverse event rates between groups and no serious adverse events overall.

STUDY CONCLUSIONS

Monthly palivizumab was safe and effective at reducing illness severity of RSV and need for hospitalization in high-risk infants.

COMMENTARY

This study was the first to demonstrate the benefits of a humanized monoclonal antibody in an infectious disease in humans, and led to IM palivizumab replacing RSV-IVIG as preferred prophylaxis in high-risk children. Ongoing debate has centered on cost–benefit analyses. Recent studies have demonstrated that the rate of RSV infection for patients born between 29 and 35 weeks' gestation approximates that of the general population,[2] leading to updated American Academy of Pediatrics (AAP) guidelines recommending the use of palivizumab only for infants <29 weeks' gestation and those with CLD of prematurity.[3]

Question

How effective is palivizumab for prophylaxis against severe RSV disease in high-risk infants?

Answer

Palivizumab significantly reduces the rate of hospitalization due to RSV infection in high-risk children, and those who are hospitalized have a milder course of illness.

References

1. Groothuis JR, Simoes EA, Levin MJ, et al. Prophylactic administration of respiratory syncytial virus immune globulin to high-risk infants and young children. The respiratory syncytial virus immune globulin study group. *N Engl J Med.* 1993;329(21):1524–1530.
2. Hall CB, Weinberg GA, Blumkin AK, et al. Respiratory syncytial virus-associated hospitalizations among children less than 24 months of age. *Pediatrics.* 2013;132(2):e341–e348.
3. American Academy of Pediatrics Committee on Infectious Diseases; American Academy of Pediatrics Bronchiolitis Guidelines Committee. Updated guidance for palivizumab prophylaxis among infants and young children at increased risk of hospitalization for respiratory syncytial virus infection. *Pediatrics.* 2014;134(2):415–420.

REDUCTION IN MOTHER-TO-CHILD TRANSMISSION OF HUMAN IMMUNODEFICIENCY VIRUS

Thomas F. Heyne ■ Chadi M. El Saleeby

Reduction of Maternal-Infant Transmission of Human Immunodeficiency Virus Type 1 With Zidovudine Treatment. Pediatric AIDS Clinical Trials Group Protocol 076 Study Group

Connor EM, Sperling RS, Gelber R, et al. *N Engl J Med.* 1994;331(18):1173–1180

BACKGROUND

Mother-to-child transmission (MTCT) of human immunodeficiency virus (HIV) is the main mode of acquisition in neonates, with approximately 20% of infants of untreated HIV-positive mothers becoming infected.[1] Acquisition risk is primarily dependent on maternal viral load and breastfeeding status; it is the highest during the last 2 trimesters of gestation, during labor and delivery, and while breastfeeding. Prior to 1994, there were no safety or efficacy studies examining the use of antiretroviral therapy (ART) to prevent MTCT.

OBJECTIVES

To assess the safety and efficacy of zidovudine (AZT) for prevention of MTCT of HIV.

METHODS

Double-blind, randomized placebo-controlled trial in 59 centers in the US and France from 1991 to 1993.

Patients

477 HIV-positive pregnant women between 14 and 34 weeks' gestation with CD4+ T-lymphocyte counts >200 and 415 live-born infants. Select exclusion criteria: prior ART, significant bone marrow, kidney or liver dysfunction, maternal or fetal anemia, other fetal anomaly.

Intervention

Comparison of placebo vs. intervention comprised of prenatal administration of AZT 100 mg PO 5 times daily and intrapartum AZT (2 mg/kg IV initially, then 1 mg/kg/h), with subsequent oral AZT (2 mg/kg every 6 hours) given to neonates for 6 weeks. Mothers and infants were followed regularly for standard checkups and toxicity monitoring. Viral cultures were obtained from infants at birth, 12, 24, and 78 weeks of life.

Outcomes

Primary outcome was infant HIV positivity on ≥1 viral culture. Secondary outcomes were adverse medication effects including anemia and thrombocytopenia.

KEY RESULTS

- At first interim analysis, 13/180 infants (8.3%, 95% CI 3.9–12.8) receiving AZT were infected vs. 40/183 infants (25.5%, 95% CI 18.4–32.5) receiving placebo, with RR reduction of 67.5% (95% CI 40.7–82.1).
- Only 1 mother reported breastfeeding her infant; this infant was not infected.
- At 6 months postpartum, there were no differences in maternal CD4 counts or progression to acquired immunodeficiency syndrome.
- Hemoglobin levels of neonates receiving AZT were mildly lower than in the placebo group (maximal difference = 1 g/dL), but they normalized by 12 weeks of age.

STUDY CONCLUSIONS

AZT given to pregnant mothers and their newborns reduced MTCT of HIV and was well tolerated, except for mild reversible anemia.

COMMENTARY

This landmark study transformed perinatal HIV care, heralding the ART era in this setting. Interim data analysis were so striking that the trial was stopped early, and AZT was offered to all patients. Today, the risk of MTCT with proper prophylaxis is significantly less than 5%, although ART resistance is an emerging concern.[2] Newer data have supported multidrug prenatal ART for optimal maternal viral load suppression. Postnatally, infants should receive prophylaxis with AZT or nevirapine, with the latter preferred in breastfed infants.[3]

Question

Is AZT safe and effective to reduce perinatal transmission of HIV?

Answer

Yes. AZZT reduced the risk of transmission by 67.5%, with minimal side effects. Newer multidrug regimens reduce this risk even further.

References

1. Cooper ER, Charurat M, Mofenson L, et al. Combination antiretroviral strategies for the treatment of pregnant HIV-1-infected women and prevention of perinatal HIV-1 transmission. *J Acquir Immune Defic Syndr.* 2002;29(5):484–494.
2. Shapiro RL, Hughes MD, Ogwu A, et al. Antiretroviral regimens in pregnancy and breast-feeding in Botswana. *N Engl J Med.* 2010;362(24):2282–2294.
3. Consolidated guidelines on the use of antiretroviral drugs for treating and preventing HIV infection: Recommendations for a public health approach. Geneva: World Health Organization; 2013. Available from: http://www.who.int/hiv/pub/guidelines/arv2013/download/en/index.html (cited 2015 July 31).

NEONATOLOGY

59. Predictors for Survival in Extreme Prematurity
60. Caffeine for Apnea of Prematurity
61. Therapeutic Hypothermia in Hypoxic-Ischemic Encephalopathy
62. Reduction of Group B Streptococcal Disease
63. Management of the Meconium-Stained Neonate
64. Bilirubin Screening in Neonates
65. Surfactant in Respiratory Distress Syndrome

PREDICTORS FOR SURVIVAL IN EXTREME PREMATURITY

Marianna Parker ■ Sara V. Bates

Intensive Care for Extreme Prematurity—Moving Beyond Gestational Age

Tyson JE, Parikh NA, Langer J, et al. *N Engl J Med.* 2008;358:1672–1681

BACKGROUND

Decisions surrounding resuscitation of and intensive care for extremely preterm infants remain challenging due to outcome variability and dating inaccuracy. In most centers, intensive care is routinely administered after 25 weeks' gestation, but practices differ for babies born at 22 to 24 weeks. Prior to this study, the effect of factors other than gestational age (GA) on survival and likelihood of severe neurodevelopmental disabilities was not well examined.

OBJECTIVES

To relate GA and other assessable perinatal factors to the likelihood of death or adverse neurologic outcomes in extremely preterm infants.

METHODS

Prospective cohort study at 19 US centers from 1998 to 2003.

Patients

4,446 infants born at 22 to 25 weeks' gestation. Select exclusion criteria: major congenital anomaly, birth weight (BW) <401 g, or BW >1,000 g or 97th percentile for GA suggesting dating inaccuracy.

Intervention

Multiple risk factors were assessed: mode of delivery, single vs. multiple birth, sex, corticosteroid treatment <7 days before delivery, race/ethnicity, and BW. Provision of intensive care was defined as initiation of mechanical ventilation. Standardized neurodevelopmental assessments were performed at corrected age of 18 to 22 months.

Outcomes

Primary outcomes were survival, survival without impairment, and survival without profound impairment (e.g., moderate/severe cerebral palsy, bilateral blindness) at corrected age of 18 to 22 months. Secondary outcomes included burden of intensive care (e.g., infant distress, resource use).

KEY RESULTS

- 83% (3,702) of all neonates received intensive care. Infants not given intensive care were more likely to have lower BW, younger GA, less exposure to prenatal corticosteroids, and vaginal birth.

- Of 4,192 study infants (94%) with available outcomes at 18 to 22 months, 49% died, 61% died/had profound impairment, and 73% died/had impairment.
- Outcomes were worse at younger GA: at 22 weeks' GA, 95% died, 98% died/had profound impairment, and 99% died/had impairment, whereas at 25 weeks' GA, 25% died, 38% died/had profound impairment, and 54% died/had impairment.
- Exposure to prenatal corticosteroids, female sex, singleton birth, and higher BW were each associated with a reduction in the risk of death or neurodevelopmental impairment, similar to gaining an extra week of GA.

STUDY CONCLUSIONS
Consideration of factors other than GA allowed for better estimation of the likelihood of death or adverse neurologic outcomes in extremely preterm infants.

COMMENTARY
This study led to the development of a multivariate prediction model to support informed decision-making regarding resuscitation and intensive care for extremely preterm neonates.[1] Continued outcomes research is vitally important, as survival rates for very low GA infants continue to increase overall, but significant inter-hospital differences in rates of survival and survival with impairment persist due to practice variability.[2] Adding to the ethical complexity is the fact that parents are often forced to confront these decisions in the context of imminent deliveries, and legal regulations vary from state to state. Resuscitation of extremely premature infants remains a highly controversial area and mandates careful consideration of all known medical data, thoughtful decision-making with the family, and clear communication with all team members.

Question
What factors other than GA are associated with reduction in adverse outcomes in extremely preterm neonates?

Answer
Prenatal corticosteroids, female sex, singleton birth, and higher BW are each independently associated with a reduction in the risk of death and neurodevelopmental impairment.

References
1. Neonatal Research Network. *Extremely Preterm Birth Outcome Data.* Bethesda, MD: National Institute for Child Health and Human Development; 2012. http://www.nichd.nih.gov/about/org/der/branches/ppb/programs/epbo/pages/epbo_case.aspx. Accessed July 28, 2015.
2. Rysavy MA, Li L, Bell EF, et al. Between-hospital variation in treatment and outcomes in extremely preterm infants. *N Engl J Med.* 2015;372(19):1801–1811.

CHAPTER 60
CAFFEINE FOR APNEA OF PREMATURITY

Marianna Parker ■ Sara V. Bates

Caffeine Therapy for Apnea of Prematurity

Schmidt B, Roberts RS, Davis P, et al. *N Engl J Med*. 2006;354(20):2112–2121

BACKGROUND

Apnea of prematurity (AOP) commonly occurs in infants born at <34 weeks' gestation. Methylxanthines (caffeine, aminophylline, theophylline) have been used for over 40 years to reduce frequency of AOP and need for mechanical ventilation in the first week. This study sought to delineate the benefits and risks of caffeine therapy in preterm neonates.

OBJECTIVES

To determine the short- and long-term efficacy and safety of caffeine therapy in very low-birth-weight (VLBW) newborns.

METHODS

Double-blind, randomized, placebo-controlled trial at multiple centers in the US, Canada, Australia, Europe, and Israel from 1999 to 2004.

Patients

2,006 infants with birth weights between 500 and 1,250 g who were considered candidates for caffeine therapy during the first 10 days of life. Select exclusion criteria: congenital anomalies with significant morbidity, previous methylxanthine treatment.

Intervention

Comparison of placebo to intervention of caffeine citrate (loading dose 20 mg/kg followed by maintenance 5 mg/kg/d and weekly weight adjustment). Maintenance dose could be increased to 10 mg/kg/d for persistent apnea. Dose was held or reduced if concern for caffeine-induced toxicity.

Outcomes

Primary outcome was a composite of death, cerebral palsy, cognitive delay, deafness, or blindness at 18 to 21 months (was under assessment at time of study's publication). Secondary short-term outcomes were the rate of bronchopulmonary dysplasia (BPD; defined as needing supplemental oxygen >36 weeks), ultrasonographic signs of brain injury, necrotizing enterocolitis (NEC), retinopathy of prematurity (ROP), and growth.

KEY RESULTS

- 36% (350/963) of neonates in the intervention group developed BPD compared with 47% (447/954) in the placebo group (OR 0.63, CI 0.52–0.76).

- Infants receiving caffeine were weaned earlier from positive airway pressure than infants given placebo (median gestational age 31 weeks vs. 32 weeks, p <0.001).
- Caffeine therapy was associated with an initial reduction in weight gain (2-week mean difference −23 g, 95% CI −32 to −13) but there was no significant difference by week 4.
- Although there was a trend toward more favorable outcomes with intervention, the rates of death, ultrasonographic signs of brain injury, and NEC did not differ significantly between the 2 groups.

STUDY CONCLUSIONS

Caffeine therapy for AOP was safe, well-tolerated, and reduced the rate of BPD in VLBW neonates.

COMMENTARY

This study altered clinical practice, leading to increased utilization of caffeine therapy soon after birth even before AOP diagnosis due to caffeine's favorable risk-benefit profile and cost effectiveness. A recent retrospective cohort study also confirmed that in very preterm neonates, early prophylactic caffeine use was associated with a reduction in the rate of patent ductus arteriosus.[1] The long-term follow-up of this trial showed a reduction in severe ROP.[2] Unfortunately, the 5-year follow-up did not show improved rates of longer-term survival without disability.[3] Future research is now investigating optimal dosing and serum concentrations of caffeine to increase efficacy while minimizing short-term side effects.

Question

What are the risks and benefits of using caffeine to treat AOP in infants?

Answer

Caffeine effectively treats apnea and reduces the rate of BPD without significant adverse effects other than short-term weight loss.

References

1. Lodha A, Seshia M, McMillan DD, et al. Association of early caffeine administration and neonatal outcomes in very preterm neonates. *JAMA Pediatr.* 2015;169(1):33–38.
2. Schmidt B, Roberts RS, Davis P, et al. Long-term effects of caffeine therapy for apnea of prematurity. *N Engl J Med.* 2007;357(19):1893–1902.
3. Schmidt B, Anderson PJ, Doyle LW, et al. Survival without disability to age 5 years after neonatal caffeine therapy for apnea of prematurity. *JAMA.* 2012;307(3):275–282.

THERAPEUTIC HYPOTHERMIA IN HYPOXIC-ISCHEMIC ENCEPHALOPATHY

Marianna Parker ■ Sara V. Bates

Whole-Body Hypothermia for Neonates With Hypoxic-Ischemic Encephalopathy

Shankaran S, Laptook AR, Ehrenkranz RA, et al. *N Engl J Med.* 2005;353(15):1574–1584

BACKGROUND

Neonatal brain injury caused by hypoxic-ischemic encephalopathy (HIE) affects 0.6% of all births.[1] 30% of infants surviving with moderate encephalopathy have significant neurologic disability and those with severe encephalopathy have even greater morbidity. Animal models had suggested that therapeutic hypothermia reduced the extent of brain injury after ischemic insult; this study sought to assess its benefits in neonates.

OBJECTIVES

To compare effects of therapeutic hypothermia vs. supportive care on mortality and disability in neonates with HIE.

METHODS

Prospective, randomized controlled trial at 15 US centers from 2000 to 2003.

Patients

208 neonates born at ≥36 weeks' gestation admitted to the neonatal intensive care unit (NICU) at ≤6 hours of age, with severe acidosis or complications requiring resuscitation at birth, and moderate or severe encephalopathy or seizures. Select exclusion criteria: major congenital anomalies, birth weight ≤1,800 g, and newborns for whom care was redirected.

Intervention

Infants in the treatment arm underwent whole-body cooling to an esophageal temperature of 33.5°C for 72 hours, followed by slow rewarming. Control group received usual intensive care. Neurologic and developmental testing was performed at 18 to 22 months of age.

Outcomes

Primary outcome was a combined endpoint of death or disability (moderate or severe).

KEY RESULTS

- Death or disability occurred in 44% (45/102) of infants in the hypothermia group vs. 62% (64/103) in the control group (risk ratio 0.72, 95% CI 0.54–0.95).
- When assessed independently, there was no statistically significant difference between the groups with respect to neonatal death.

- Survivors who underwent hypothermia did not have an increase in major disability. Cerebral palsy occurred in 19% (15/77) of infants receiving hypothermia vs. 30% (19/64) in control group (risk ratio 0.68, 95% CI 0.38–1.22).
- The incidence of serious adverse events was similar in both groups.

STUDY CONCLUSIONS
Whole-body hypothermia was safe and effective in reducing the combined risk of death or disability in infants with moderate or severe HIE.

COMMENTARY
This was one of the first trials demonstrating the safety and efficacy of whole-body hypothermia as treatment for neonatal HIE. Subsequent studies supported these findings, establishing therapeutic hypothermia as the current standard of care.[2] Subgroup analyses in this study population showed that moderately affected infants had larger improvements in outcomes than those who were more severely affected. Further research, however, did not show reduction in death from longer or deeper cooling.[3] Studies are currently underway to determine potential benefits of hypothermia in infants outside the initial inclusion criteria (gestational age <36 weeks, time of arrival >6 hours), as well as to assess xenon and topiramate as possible adjuvant therapies.[4]

Question
Should therapeutic hypothermia be used as treatment for infants with HIE?

Answer
Yes, infants at a gestational age ≥36 weeks with perinatal depression and moderate-to-severe encephalopathy should be treated with hypothermia within 6 hours to reduce death or disability. Infants outside this narrow group may be considered for treatment with hypothermia on a case-by-case basis.

References
1. Lai MC, Yang SN. Perinatal hypoxic-ischemic encephalopathy. *J Biomed Biotechnol.* 2011;2011:609813.
2. Edwards AD, Brocklehurst P, Gunn AJ, et al. Neurological outcomes at 18 months of age after moderate hypothermia for perinatal hypoxic ischaemic encephalopathy: Synthesis and meta-analysis of the trial data. *BMJ.* 2010;340:c363.
3. Shankaran S, Laptook AR, Pappas A, et al. Effect of depth and duration of cooling on deaths in the NICU among neonates with hypoxic ischemic encephalopathy: A randomized clinical trial. *JAMA.* 2014;312(24):2629–2639.
4. Committee on Fetus and Newborn, Papile LA, Baley JE, et al. Hypothermia and neonatal encephalopathy. *Pediatrics.* 2014;133(6):1146–1150.

CHAPTER 62

REDUCTION OF GROUP B STREPTOCOCCAL DISEASE

Marianna Parker ■ Sara V. Bates

A Population-based Comparison of Strategies to Prevent Early-Onset Group B Streptococcal Disease in Neonates

Schrag SJ, Zell ER, Lynfield R, et al. *New Engl J Med.* 2002;347(4):233–239

BACKGROUND

Perinatal group B streptococcal (GBS) infections remain a leading cause of illness and death among newborns in the United States, affecting about 1:3,000 live births.[1] In 1996, both the American Congress of Obstetricians and Gynecologists and American Academy of Pediatrics guidelines recommended 1 of 2 approaches for intrapartum antibiotic prophylaxis: universal screening or risk-based. However, the comparative effectiveness of these 2 strategies had not been well analyzed prior to this study.

OBJECTIVES

To evaluate the effectiveness of universal screening compared with the risk-based approach in preventing early-onset GBS disease.

METHODS

Retrospective cohort study in 8 geographic areas in the US from 1998 to 1999.

Patients

5,144 neonates randomly sampled from areas with active surveillance for GBS infection, including all cases of early-onset disease (occurring at <7 days old).

Intervention

Comparison of universal screening (all women screened for GBS carriage with rectovaginal culture between 35 and 37 weeks' gestation with intrapartum antibiotic prophylaxis [IAP] offered to carriers) with the risk-based approach (women presenting in labor with clinical risk factors for GBS transmission [e.g., fever, prolonged rupture of membranes, preterm delivery] offered IAP).

Outcomes

Primary outcome was risk of early-onset GBS disease in the screening group relative to the risk-based group.

KEY RESULTS

- 52% (2,628/5,144) of mothers were screened for GBS before delivery.
- There were 312 cases of early-onset GBS disease; of these, 34.3% of mothers had been screened for GBS before delivery.

- 62% (195/312) of women whose newborns had early-onset GBS did not have clinical risk factors for disease transmission (i.e., <37 weeks' gestation, rupture of membranes ≥18 hours before delivery, intrapartum fever ≥38°C, GBS bacteriuria, previous infant with GBS).
- Risk of early-onset disease was significantly lower among infants of universally screened women than those in the risk-based screening group (adjusted RR 0.46, 95% CI 0.36–0.60).

STUDY CONCLUSIONS

Universal screening for GBS during pregnancy prevented more cases of early-onset disease than a risk-based approach, even when controlled for known risk factors.

COMMENTARY

This study informed the updated 2002 Centers for Disease Control and Prevention guidelines recommending universal GBS screening at 35 to 37 weeks' gestation. Since its adoption, the use of IAP in GBS-positive women has reduced the incidence of early-onset disease by 33%.[2] However, universal screening remains controversial due to the lack of randomized trials assessing the effect on infant morbidity and mortality.[1] There are also concerns regarding IAP safety, antimicrobial resistance, and increased incidence of non-GBS neonatal pathogens. Furthermore, the optimal timing of culture data remains unclear since GBS colonization status can change throughout pregnancy.[2] This has propelled development of rapid diagnostics including real-time PCR to test for GBS carriage at labor onset. It is important to recognize that universal screening and IAP have had no effect on late-onset GBS disease or in utero disease (including stillbirths and miscarriages).[2] Even with improved screening technologies, GBS disease is unlikely to be eliminated until the development of an effective GBS vaccine.

Question

Is universal GBS screening in pregnant women or a risk-based approach more effective at preventing early-onset neonatal disease?

Answer

Universal screening at 35 to 37 weeks' gestation to guide the use of intrapartum antibiotic prophylaxis is more effective than risk-based screening at preventing early-onset neonatal GBS.

References

1. Puopolo KM, Madoff LC, Eichenwald EC. Early-onset group B streptococcal disease in the era of maternal screening. *Pediatrics.* 2005;115(5):1240–1246.
2. Verani JR, McGee L, Schrag SJ, et al. Prevention of perinatal group B streptococcal disease–revised guidelines from CDC, 2010. *MMWR Recomm Rep.* 2010;59(RR-10):1–36.

<tr><td rowspan="3" style="background:#000;color:#fff;">CHAPTER 63</td><td rowspan="3">MANAGEMENT OF THE MECONIUM-STAINED NEONATE</td></tr>
</table>

MANAGEMENT OF THE MECONIUM-STAINED NEONATE

CHAPTER 63

Marianna Parker ■ Sara V. Bates

Delivery Room Management of the Apparently Vigorous Meconium-Stained Neonate: Results of the Multicenter, International Collaborative Trial

Wiswell TE, Gannon CM, Jacob J, et al. *Pediatrics.* 2000;105(1 Pt 1):1–7

BACKGROUND

Meconium-stained amniotic fluid (MSAF) is noted in ~13% of deliveries, with some infants developing meconium aspiration syndrome (MAS). Observational studies from the 1970s suggested that intubation and suctioning at delivery could reduce development of MAS and decrease mortality, leading to routine intubation and suctioning for all infants born through MSAF. In the late 1980s, however, deleterious effects were noted with routine suctioning of vigorous neonates.[1] This study was the first large randomized trial assessing whether the tracheal suctioning technique prevented MAS.

OBJECTIVES

To assess whether intubation and suctioning of vigorous, meconium-stained neonates would reduce the incidence of MAS compared to routine delivery room care, and to evaluate the complication rate of this approach.

METHODS

Prospective randomized controlled trial in 12 centers in the United States, Argentina, and Paraguay from 1995 to 1997.

Patients

2,094 neonates ≥37 weeks' gestation born through MSAF with HR >100, spontaneous respirations, and good tone immediately after birth. Select exclusion criteria: lack of apparent vigor.

Intervention

Infants in the intervention group (INT) were intubated immediately after assessment of vigor with 1 to 5 seconds of suctioning during endotracheal tube withdrawal. If endotracheal meconium was suctioned, the procedure was repeated until no further MSAF was withdrawn. Infants assigned to expectant management (EXP) had routine delivery room care.

Outcomes

Primary outcomes were the incidence of respiratory distress, MAS, and intubation complications.

KEY RESULTS

- There was no significant difference in MAS incidence between the 2 groups (3.2% INT vs. 2.7% EXP).
- 149 (7.1%) infants subsequently developed respiratory distress. 62 (3%) had MAS but 87 (4.2%) were found to have other disorders (e.g., transient tachypnea of the newborn).
- Of 1,092 successfully intubated infants, 42 (3.8%) had a total of 51 complications including bradycardia ($n = 26$), stridor/hoarseness ($n = 14$), laryngospasm ($n = 6$), apnea ($n = 2$), bleeding ($n = 2$), and cyanosis ($n = 2$). Most of these complications were transient and mild.

STUDY CONCLUSIONS

Compared with expectant management, intubation and suctioning of the apparently vigorous meconium-stained infant was well tolerated, but did not decrease the incidence of MAS or other respiratory disorders.

COMMENTARY

Delivery room management of infants born through MSAF has evolved over the past several decades. This study informed current perinatal care guidelines which no longer recommend routine intubation and suctioning of vigorous meconium-stained infants. Obstetric management has also evolved in tandem; oral and nasopharyngeal suctioning at the perineum is no longer recommended after a 2004 trial demonstrated no decrease in MAS incidence or severity.[2] Of note, this study lacked informed consent from participants' families, as the researchers stated that both management strategies (universal vs. selective intubation) were widely accepted as standards of care. In addition, there were inherent difficulties obtaining consent due to maternal discomfort and timing of MSAF identification. Currently, the focus of debate is whether depressed infants born through MSAF also still need to be routinely intubated and suctioned, as MAS is increasingly thought to develop as a result of an in utero event, with the insult having already occurred by the time of delivery.

Question

Should meconium-stained infants be routinely intubated and suctioned at delivery?

Answer

No, vigorous meconium-stained infants do not benefit from additional intervention and do well with expectant management.

References

1. Linder N, Aranda JV, Tsur M, et al. Need for endotracheal intubation and suction in meconium-stained neonates. *J Pediatr.* 1988;112(4):613–615.
2. Vain NE, Szyld EG, Prudent LM, et al. Oropharyngeal and nasopharyngeal suctioning of meconium-stained neonates before delivery of their shoulders: Multicentre, randomised controlled trial. *Lancet.* 2004;364(9434):597–602.

CHAPTER 64

BILIRUBIN SCREENING IN NEONATES

Rebecca Cook ■ Sara V. Bates

Predictive Ability of a Predischarge Hour-Specific Serum Bilirubin for Subsequent Significant Hyperbilirubinemia in Healthy Term and Near-Term Newborns

Bhutani VK, Johnson L, Sivieri EM. *Pediatrics.* 1999;103(1):6–14

BACKGROUND

Extreme hyperbilirubinemia has been estimated to occur in 25:100,000 term and near-term neonates, with approximately one-third developing kernicterus, which can be associated with hearing loss, encephalopathy, and cerebral palsy.[1] Neurotoxicity at time of presentation with extreme hyperbilirubinemia is more common in infants who have been discharged home. As physical examination alone is not reliable at recognizing significant neonatal jaundice, identifying newborns at high risk of developing significant hyperbilirubinemia could improve outcomes by allowing closer follow-up after discharge and appropriate treatment before progression. This study sought to use predischarge total serum bilirubin (TSB) to identify infants at low, intermediate, and high risk of significant neonatal jaundice post-discharge.

OBJECTIVES

To assess the predictive ability of a universal predischarge TSB screening to identify healthy term and near-term infants at risk for development of post-discharge significant hyperbilirubinemia.

METHODS

Prospective cohort study in a single US academic center from 1993 to 1997.

Patients

2,840 term and near-term newborns with appropriate birth weight for gestational age (≥2,000 g for ≥36 weeks' gestation and ≥2,500 g for 35 to 36 weeks' gestation). Select exclusion criteria: intensive care unit admission, Coombs positivity, phototherapy before 60 hours of life, or no post-discharge TSB.

Intervention

TSB measurement pre-discharge, between 24 and 48 hours post-discharge and when indicated based on phototherapy guidelines. These data were then used to create a risk-prediction nomogram based on the frequency of subsequent significant hyperbilirubinemia. Clinical and demographic risk factors for hyperbilirubinemia were also recorded.

Outcomes

Primary outcome was clinically significant hyperbilirubinemia in the high-risk zone (post-discharge TSB value ≥95th percentile).

KEY RESULTS

- 49.5% of newborns were exclusively breastfed, 60% were partially breastfed, and 4.1% of the study population required phototherapy.
- 6% (172/2,840) of neonates had a high-risk pre-discharge TSB, 32% (912/2,840) had an intermediate-risk pre-discharge TSB, and 61.8% (1,756/2,840) had a low-risk pre-discharge TSB.
- 39.5% of neonates with a high-risk pre-discharge TSB also had a high-risk post-discharge TSB (LR = 14.08, 54% sensitivity, 96.2% specificity).
- 6.4% of newborns in the intermediate-risk zone pre-discharge crossed into the high-risk zone after discharge.
- No neonates with a low-risk pre-discharge TSB developed clinically significant hyperbilirubinemia post-discharge (LR = 0, 100% sensitivity, 64.7% specificity).
- See Figure 64.1.

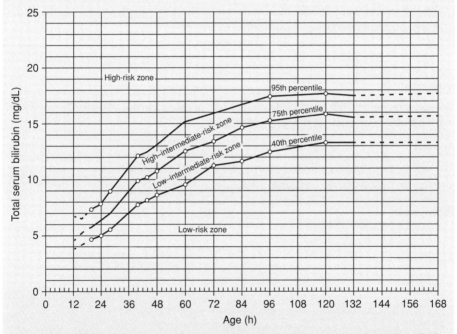

Figure 64.1 Risk designation of term and near-term well newborns based on their hour-specific serum bilirubin values. (From Bhutani VK, Johnson L, Sivieri EM. Predictive ability of a predischarge hour-specific serum bilirubin for subsequent significant hyperbilirubinemia in healthy term and near-term newborns. *Pediatrics.* 1999;103(1):6–14.)

STUDY CONCLUSIONS

Pre-discharge TSB predicted whether a newborn was at high, intermediate, or low risk for clinically significant hyperbilirubinemia. Universal screening allows focus of resources and follow-up for those at highest risk.

COMMENTARY

The "Bhutani nomogram" (see Fig. 64.1) developed from these data in a diverse population was a landmark development in newborn medicine and now serves as the standard of care in routine risk assessment of severe hyperbilirubinemia in well newborns.[2] Since its development, additional risk factors have been identified, including gestational age and exclusive breastfeeding. Those infants with initial predischarge TSB in the high- and high–intermediate-risk zones should have repeat testing, typically before discharge, and those at low-intermediate risk should have close outpatient follow-up. Transcutaneous bilirubin is often used to simplify screening, but is not a precise proxy for TSB which should be checked whenever therapy is being considered.

Question

Can pre-discharge TSB adequately predict risk of development of clinically significant hyperbilirubinemia post-discharge in neonates?

Answer

For healthy term or near-term newborns, the Bhutani nomogram can be used to stratify risk based on pre-discharge TSB.

References

1. Ebbesen F, Andersson C, Verder H, et al. Extreme hyperbilirubinaemia in term and near-term infants in Denmark. *Acta Paediatr.* 2005;94(1):59–64.
2. American Academy of Pediatrics Subcommittee on Hyperbilirubinemia. Management of hyperbilirubinemia in the newborn infant 35 or more weeks of gestation. *Pediatrics.* 2004;114(1):297–316.

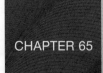

SURFACTANT IN RESPIRATORY DISTRESS SYNDROME

CHAPTER 65

Rebecca Cook ■ Sara V. Bates

Artificial Surfactant Therapy in Hyaline-Membrane Disease

Fujiwara T, Maeta H, Chida S, et al. *Lancet.* 1980;1(8159):55–59

BACKGROUND

Surfactant, a complex lipoprotein, reduces surface tension in pulmonary alveoli. Its deficiency leads to widespread atelectasis, barotrauma, inflammation, and tissue damage that cause respiratory distress syndrome (RDS) in preterm and low-birth-weight infants. Before the development of surfactant therapy, RDS affected 40% to 60% of infants with birth weight (BW) 500 to 1,500 g, with ≥20% mortality.[1] This was the first human study exploring whether treatment with artificial surfactant improved outcomes in neonates with severe RDS.

OBJECTIVES

To assess the impact of artificial surfactant delivery on subsequent need for ventilation and clinical outcomes in preterm neonates.

METHODS

Prospective cohort study in a single center in Japan in 1979.

Patients

10 neonates (mean gestational age 30.2 weeks, mean BW 1,152 g) admitted to a neonatal intensive care unit (NICU) with severe RDS who were not improving with initial intubation and ventilation.

Intervention

Administration of 150 μmol/kg of artificial surfactant at an average of 12 hours of life.

Outcomes

NICU clinical course including fraction of inspired oxygen (FiO_2), gas exchange, and length of artificial ventilation.

KEY RESULTS

- Within 6 hours of surfactant administration, there were improvements in mean blood pressure (increased from 37 ± 5 to 59 ± 4 mm Hg, p <0.02); FiO_2 (decreased from 0.80 ± 0.07 to 0.40 ± 0.05, p <0.01); and mean peak inspiratory pressure (decreased from 30 ± 2 to 22 ± 2 cm H_2O, p <0.02).
- The alveolar-arterial oxygen difference decreased after surfactant administration (474 ± 49 to 189 ± 29 [p <0.005] after 3 hours, 120 ± 18 [p <0.001] after 30 hours).

- Radiographic evidence of RDS resolved on average only 6 hours after administration of surfactant.
- The mean total duration of endotracheal intubation was 13 ± 3.3 days.
- 2 of 10 infants died from complications not related to RDS; there were no observed complications directly related to artificial surfactant delivery.

STUDY CONCLUSIONS

In neonates with RDS, surfactant therapy significantly improved gas exchange, ventilation, and radiographic resolution of infiltrates.

COMMENTARY

This ground-breaking study led to the widespread use of surfactant for severe RDS and changed neonatology practice. While this small cohort had no long-term follow-up, subsequent data have demonstrated improved mortality and morbidity with surfactant use. More than 30 years later, however, the criteria for administration, optimal timing, dose, and delivery method are still debated. Both the American Academy of Pediatrics and the European consensus guidelines endorse the early use of surfactant in premature infants with RDS, but its role as a prophylactic agent during intubation in the delivery room is increasingly under scrutiny given improving outcomes with the use of continuous positive airway pressure (CPAP) alone. In addition, the role of exogenous surfactant in infants with other pulmonary conditions associated with surfactant deficiency (such as lung hypoplasia, meconium aspiration syndrome, and respiratory distress associated with maternal diabetes) continues to be explored.[2]

Question

Does surfactant administration improve lung function in preterm neonates with RDS?

Answer

Yes, surfactant administration improves respiratory function in preterm newborns. Additional indications for use are currently under exploration.

References
1. Liechty EA, Donovan E, Purohit D, et al. Reduction of neonatal mortality after multiple doses of bovine surfactant in low birth weight neonates with respiratory distress syndrome. *Pediatrics.* 1991;88(1):19–28.
2. Lopez E, Gascoin G, Flamant C, et al. Exogenous surfactant therapy in 2013: What is next? Who, when and how should we treat newborn infants in the future? *BMC Pediatr.* 2013;13:165.

NEUROLOGY

66. Seizure Recurrence After Withdrawal of Antiepileptic Drugs
67. Developmental Outcomes After Preterm Births
68. Serious Intracranial Pathology in Chronic Headache
69. Amitryptiline in Migraine Prophylaxis
70. Risk of Unprovoked Seizures After Febrile Seizures

SEIZURE RECURRENCE AFTER WITHDRAWAL OF ANTIEPILEPTIC DRUGS

Melissa A. Walker ■ Kevin J. Staley

Recurrence Risk After Withdrawal of Antiepileptic Drugs in Children With Epilepsy: A Prospective Study

Ramos-Lizana J, Aguirre-Rodríguez J, Aguilera-López P, et al. *Eur J Paediatr Neurol.* 2010;14(2):116–124

BACKGROUND

Many children will outgrow epilepsy and no longer need antiepileptic drugs (AED), which have many potential side effects and interactions. However, previous studies provided little guidance on when AED monotherapy may be stopped without increasing risk of recurrent seizure.[1] This study analyzed remission after cessation of AEDs per current practice guidelines.

OBJECTIVES

To determine seizure recurrence risk and prognostic factors predicting relapse in children with epilepsy after AED withdrawal.

METHODS

Prospective, observational trial at a single center in Spain from 1994 to 2004.

Patients

353 children ages 0 to 13 years with a history of ≥2 unprovoked seizures separated by ≥24 hours. Select exclusion criteria: exclusive neonatal seizures, inborn error of metabolism, neurodegenerative disorder.

Intervention

AEDs were stopped after patients had been in remission ≥2 years. Patients were then followed by personal interview for 1 to 3 years and telephone for ≥5 years. In addition, baseline and follow-up EEGs and baseline imaging were reviewed when available.

Outcomes

Primary outcome was seizure recurrence risk after 2 years off AEDs.

KEY RESULTS

- 90% (309/343) of children were initially treated with AEDs. 77% (238/309) of those children achieved remission (mean seizure-free time 2.16 ± 0.6 years), of whom 216 then consented to AED withdrawal.
- Seizure recurrence risk after AED withdrawal was 23% at 2 years (95% CI 17–29) and 28% at 5 years (95% CI 22–34).

- An increase in risk of seizure recurrence was noted with epilepsy secondary to an acquired insult (41%, 85% CI 28–54), prior febrile seizures (p <0.05), prior neonatal seizures (p <0.05), global developmental delay (p <0.05), abnormal neuroimaging (p <0.05), and particular seizure types predictive of increased recurrence risk (e.g., nonabsence idiopathic generalized epilepsy, cryptogenic partial seizures, etc.).

STUDY CONCLUSIONS

In all children with epilepsy, recurrent seizure risk after withdrawal of AEDs was relatively low. The etiology of an individual's epilepsy was the primary predictor.

COMMENTARY

This study supported earlier data from 1996 guidelines, suggesting that predictors of successful AED cessation were: no seizures for 2 to 5 years, a single type of partial or primary generalized tonic–clonic seizures, normal physical examination and intelligence quotient, and normalization of EEG on treatment.[2] These parameters, considered in conjunction with individual patient variables (e.g., driving, activities, and living situation) should guide the decision to attempt AED taper. A 2015 Cochrane review confirmed a 2-year seizure-free interval before AED taper, although it notes insufficient evidence in children with generalized seizures.[3] Given the increased risk of seizure recurrence associated with particular syndromes and expansion of diagnostic testing capabilities, future patient education will likely incorporate the results of genetic studies.

Question

When is it safe to consider stopping AEDs in children with epilepsy in remission?

Answer

Children with epilepsy in remission are unlikely to experience seizure recurrence after AED withdrawal if they have been seizure free for 2 years and have specific low-risk epilepsy syndromes.

References

1. Hixson JD. Stopping antiepileptic drugs: When and why? *Curr Treat Options Neurol.* 2010;12(5):434–442.
2. Practice parameter: A guideline for discontinuing antiepileptic drugs in seizure-free patients–summary statement. Report of the Quality Standards Subcommittee of the American Academy of Neurology. *Neurology.* 1996;47(2):600–602.
3. Strozzi I, Nolan SJ, Sperling MR, et al. Early versus late antiepileptic drug withdrawal for people with epilepsy in remission. *Cochrane Database Syst Rev.* 2015;2:CD001902.

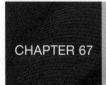

DEVELOPMENTAL OUTCOMES AFTER PRETERM BIRTHS

CHAPTER 67

Melissa A. Walker ■ Kevin J. Staley

Lasting Effects of Preterm Birth and Neonatal Brain Hemorrhage at 12 Years of Age
Luu TM, Ment LR, Schneider KC, et al. *Pediatrics*. 2009;123(3):1037–1044

BACKGROUND

Preterm children with normal intelligence have higher rates of neurodevelopmental disabilities compared to their term peers; high-grade intraventricular hemorrhages (IVHs) can lead to additional sequelae in these children.[1] However, the majority of outcome data was from infants born in the late 1970s to early 1980s. Given interval improvements in neonatal care including administration of prenatal steroids and surfactant with resultant improved survival, this study sought to assess the effect of preterm birth on current long-term developmental outcomes.

OBJECTIVES

To describe cognitive, language, and behavioral outcomes of preterm children at 12 years of age.

METHODS

Prospective observational study at 3 US centers of children born between 1989 and 1992.

Patients

375 children age 12 years born prematurely with very low birth weight (600 to 1,250 g) cared for in the neonatal intensive care unit and 111 children born at full term who served as matched controls. Select exclusion criteria: presence of grade 3–4 IVH, periventricular leukomalacia, or severe ventriculomegaly on cranial ultrasound.

Intervention

Clinical data were reviewed for all patients. Children were assessed by neuropsychometric testing, neurologic examination, and interviews regarding educational needs.

Outcomes

Primary outcome was intelligence quotient (IQ) by the Wechsler Intelligence Scale for Children-III. Secondary outcomes were scores of neurodevelopmental function.

KEY RESULTS

- Children born preterm had lower mean full scale (87.9 vs. 103.8), verbal (90.8 vs. 103.9), and performance IQs (86.8 vs. 103.1) as compared to controls.
- The majority of preterm children free of neonatal brain injury (88%) and with brain injury (68%) were enrolled in a regular classroom. However, preterm children

required more school services, with greatest needs seen in those with brain injury (76% with brain injury; 44% without brain injury; 16% of controls).
- Preterm children were 5 times more likely to have ≥1 behavioral problem as compared to term controls.
- On multivariate analysis, the strongest predictor of lower intelligence scores was severe neonatal brain injury (grade 3–4 IVH, periventricular leukomalacia, or ≥ grade 2 ventriculomegaly), though there was also an association with minority status. Predictors of better outcome included prenatal steroids, higher maternal education, and 2-parent family.

STUDY CONCLUSIONS
Preterm, very low-birth-weight infants, particularly those with history of brain injury, had lower IQ scores and required increased school services at age 12 as compared to control patients born at term.

COMMENTARY
This work constitutes an important contribution, clearly indicating that both prematurity-associated IVH and prematurity alone (without neuroanatomic insult) have significant long-term impacts on neurodevelopment. Notably, these findings were evident even in the era of advanced neonatal intensive care including prenatal steroids and surfactant. Following this large-scale study with well-matched controls, additional work has explored the specific effects of IVH on neurodevelopmental outcomes and has confirmed similar findings.[1,2]

Question
Do prematurity and neonatal brain injury have long-term impacts on intelligence?

Answer
Yes, even in the setting of optimal neonatal care, both IVH and prematurity have discernible, adverse effects on neurodevelopmental outcomes, behavior, and school performance.

References
1. Bassan H, Limperopoulos C, Visconti K, et al. Neurodevelopmental outcome in survivors of periventricular hemorrhagic infarction. *Pediatrics.* 2007;120(4):785–792.
2. Patra K, Wilson-Costello D, Taylor HG, et al. Grades I-II intraventricular hemorrhage in extremely low birth weight infants: Effects on neurodevelopment. *J Pediatr.* 2006;149(2):169–173.

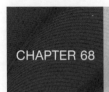

SERIOUS INTRACRANIAL PATHOLOGY IN CHRONIC HEADACHE

CHAPTER 68

Melissa A. Walker ■ Kevin J. Staley

Serious Neurological Disorders in Children With Chronic Headache
Abu-Arafeh I, Macleod S. *Arch Dis Child.* 2005;90:937–940

BACKGROUND

The prevalence of headache in children worldwide is estimated to be roughly 60%. Only 1:10 pediatric patients with intracranial tumors will present with isolated headache;[1] however, the risk of missing a potentially life-threatening diagnosis can lead to overuse of imaging in headache evaluation. Several prior studies evaluating the role of neuroimaging in children with headache did not demonstrate additional benefit from routine use of MRI or CT screening in identifying intracranial abnormalities not predicted by clinical examination.[2]

OBJECTIVES

To assess the prevalence of serious neurologic disorders (clinically anticipated and unanticipated) in children presenting with isolated headache.

METHODS

Prospective observational study conducted in a single UK pediatric headache clinic from 1996 to 2003.

Patients

815 children ages 1 to 18 years referred to the headache clinic. Select exclusion criteria: none.

Intervention

Children were prospectively assessed by history, physical, and neurologic examination with subsequent neuroimaging performed if indicated. Follow-up with headache diaries was done for variable amounts of time.

Outcomes

Primary outcome was incidence of serious intracranial pathology.

KEY RESULTS

- Mean duration of headache was 21.2 months (SD 21.2).
- Of 815 children seen, 142 (17.5%) had neuroimaging by CT, MRI, or both, with 89 (73%) of these having imaging prior to referral.
- Headache in 3 children (0.37%, 95% CI 0.08–1.1) was caused by active intracranial pathology: 2 with brain tumors and 1 with sagittal sinus thrombosis. Diagnosis of one of the brain tumors and the sinus thrombosis was clinically predicted prior to imaging.

STUDY CONCLUSIONS

Serious intracranial conditions in children presenting with isolated chronic headache were rare, and the majority were identified with careful history and clinical examination prior to neuroimaging.

COMMENTARY

This work strengthens prior evidence that serious intracranial pathology in children with isolated chronic headache is rare (even in a subspecialty clinic where more severe cases may be seen) and that neuroimaging is not superior to clinical assessment in identifying patients with serious intracranial pathology. Headaches of shorter duration (2 to 4 months) have a higher incidence of association with intracranial pathology, although they are almost all (96%) accompanied by seizures or an abnormal neurologic examination, limiting their inclusion in isolated chronic headache cohorts.[3] Thus in neurologically normal children, the longer that headache remains the only symptom, the less useful imaging will be. Imaging should be considered in cases where the neurologic examination is abnormal or the history includes other conditions predisposing the patient to serious intracranial pathology (e.g., hemiplegic migraines). Careful follow-up is crucial; serious intracranial pathology, while unlikely, is never absolutely exonerated by a single evaluation as symptoms and pathologies can both evolve and progress.

Question

How common is serious intracranial pathology in children with chronic isolated headache?

Answer

Isolated chronic headache in children is rarely the result of serious intracranial pathology particularly when present for a long duration; neuroimaging should be considered when there are abnormal findings on the clinical examination or predisposing conditions on history.

References

1. Abu-Arafeh I, Razak S, Sivaraman B, et al. Prevalence of headache and migraine in children and adolescents: A systematic review of population-based studies. *Dev Med Child Neurol.* 2010;52(12):1088–1097.
2. Lewis DW, Dorbad D. The utility of neuroimaging in the evaluation of children with migraine or chronic daily headache who have normal neurological examinations. *Headache.* 2000;40(8):629–632.
3. Wilne SH, Ferris RC, Nathwani A, et al. The presenting features of brain tumors: A review of 200 cases. *Arch Dis Child.* 2006;91(6):502–506.

CHAPTER 69

AMITRIPTYLINE IN MIGRAINE PROPHYLAXIS

Melissa A. Walker ■ Kevin J. Staley

Effectiveness of Amitriptyline in the Prophylactic Management of Childhood Headaches
Hershey AD, Powers SW, Bentti AL, et al. *Headache.* 2000;40(7):539–549

BACKGROUND

Worldwide prevalence of headache in children is approximately 60%, with significant associated morbidity, including school absenteeism and impaired interactions with family and peers.[1,2] In the 1970s, several studies established amitriptyline as one of the more effective and better-tolerated adult migraine prophylactic agents, with an average efficacy of 42%. This was the first large-scale pediatric study.

OBJECTIVES

To assess the effectiveness of amitriptyline for pediatric headache prophylaxis.

METHODS

Prospective observational study in a single outpatient headache center from 1997 to 1999.

Patients

192 school-age patients who reported >3 headaches per month. Select exclusion criteria: prior prophylaxis, initiation of another medication.

Intervention

Amitriptyline was started at 0.25 mg/kg nightly (slowly titrated to 1 mg/kg) and continued until development of intolerable side effects, lack of adherence, lack of benefit at 3 months, or successful treatment for 4 to 6 months (reduced headache frequency to ≤2/month). Baseline and follow-up characterization of headaches (using a standardized questionnaire) and school attendance were recorded at regularly scheduled visits.

Outcomes

Primary outcomes were the frequency, duration, severity, and perception of headaches, and school days missed.

KEY RESULTS

- 84.2% (162/192) of children reported subjective improvement in headache at the initial follow-up visit.
- Treated children demonstrated reductions in headache frequency (17.1 ± 10.1 days/month down to 9.2 ± 10, p <0.001), duration (11.5 ± 15 hours down to 6.3 ± 11.1), and school days missed (5.3 ± 10 down to 1.3 ± 3.1, p <0.001) at first return visit.

- Only 20.8% (40/192) of patients returned for a fourth visit, at which time 82.5% reported subjective improvement, with headache occurrence on 7.1 ± 10.3 days/month ($p < 0.001$).

STUDY CONCLUSIONS

A daily dose of 1 mg/kg amitriptyline was an effective prophylactic medication for children with >3 headaches per month.

COMMENTARY

This study, along with other small pediatric studies comparing tricyclic antidepressants and other agents (e.g., topiramate and propranolol) for headache prophylaxis, informed the 2004 American Academy of Neurology practice recommendations.[2] Currently, there are still no completed placebo-controlled trials of individual agents or comparison studies to definitively recommend any single prophylactic agent. Practitioners must therefore continue to exercise clinical judgment in selecting medications, often directed by side effect profiles. Limitations of this study include lack of a control group (relevant as many patients improve without targeted therapy), inclusion of patients with both migrainous and non-migrainous headaches, use of biobehavioral treatment in addition to amitriptyline, and utilization of higher pediatric doses than the typical 5 to 10 mg nightly. The National Institutes of Health-sponsored Childhood and Adolescent Migraine Prevention (CHAMP) study is currently ongoing, aiming to provide Level 1 evidence for the effectiveness of both amitriptyline and topiramate for migraine prophylaxis in children and adolescents.[3]

Question

Is amitriptyline effective prophylaxis for pediatric headaches?

Answer

Yes, although there was no control group for comparison, amitriptyline 1 mg/kg nightly was shown to decrease frequency and duration of headaches as well as school absenteeism.

References

1. Abu-Arafeh I, Razak S, Sivaraman B, et al. Prevalence of headache and migraine in children and adolescents: A systematic review of population-based studies. *Dev Med Child Neurol.* 2010;52(12):1088–1097.
2. Lewis D, Ashwal S, Hershey A, et al. Practice parameter: Pharmacological treatment of migraine headache in children and adolescents: Report of the American Academy of Neurology Quality Standards Subcommittee and the Practice Committee of the Child Neurology Society. *Neurology.* 2004;63(12):2215–2224.
3. Hershey AD, Powers SW, Coffey CS, et al. Childhood and Adolescent Migraine Prevention (CHAMP) study: A double-blinded, placebo-controlled, comparative effectiveness study of amitriptyline, topiramate, and placebo in the prevention of childhood and adolescent migraine. *Headache.* 2013;53(5):799–816.

RISK OF UNPROVOKED SEIZURES AFTER FEBRILE SEIZURES

Melissa A. Walker ■ Kevin J. Staley

Factors Prognostic of Unprovoked Seizures After Febrile Convulsions

Annegers JF, Hauser WA, Shirts SB, et al. *N Engl J Med.* 1987;316(9):493–498

BACKGROUND

It had been unknown how long the risk of unprovoked seizure after febrile seizure persisted, or if semiology (e.g., focal features) was prognostic. Groups had found the risk of subsequent unprovoked seizure as low as 2.5% after simple febrile seizures and as high as 17% after complex febrile seizures.[1] This study was the first to follow patients into adulthood, and examine independent risk factors for future unprovoked seizures.

OBJECTIVES

To determine features associated with risk of future unprovoked seizures in children with a prior febrile seizure.

METHODS

Population-based, prospective cohort study using data from a single US city from 1935 to 1979.

Patients

687 children with febrile seizures without history of prior unprovoked seizure. Select exclusion criteria: intelligence quotient (IQ) <70, cerebral palsy, central nervous system infection.

Intervention

Demographic, clinical, and family data were collected for patients at the time of first febrile seizure. Medical records were then subsequently followed until occurrence of unprovoked seizure, out-of-area move, or end of study, for a total of >10,000 person-years (average 18 years/patient).

Outcomes

Primary outcome was development of unprovoked, afebrile seizures. Secondary outcomes were risk factors associated with subsequent seizure occurrence and seizure type.

KEY RESULTS

- Children with any febrile seizures had an average 7% risk of later unprovoked seizures. There was a higher risk if the initial seizure had focality (RR 3.6, 95% CI 1.4–9.1), lasted ≥30 minutes (RR 2.8, 95% CI 1.0–7.8), or if there was ≥1 seizure in a 24-hour period (RR 2.8, 95% CI 1.3–6).

- Children experiencing simple febrile seizures had a 2.4% risk of unprovoked seizures through age 25, while those with complex features (but no other risk factors) had an 8% risk (95% CI 3–19).
- Cumulative risk of unprovoked seizure increased with increasing number of complex features: there was a 49% risk in children with focal features, repeated episodes, and prolonged duration.

STUDY CONCLUSIONS

In long-term follow-up, the absolute risk of subsequent unprovoked seizures in children with febrile seizures was low, but increased with the presence of complex features.

COMMENTARY

Strengths of this study include its large power, long duration, and prospective design. The impact of potentially important confounders was minimized by the study's location in a single city, as well as exclusion of patients with multiple concomitant conditions (e.g., CNS infection, trauma, cerebral palsy, low IQ), though these factors limit the study's generalizability. Additionally, as patients with neonatal seizures were included, many important underlying conditions increasing the risk of future seizures such as metabolic and genetic disorders, and hypoxic/ischemic injury were not specifically identified. Importantly, this study examined the risk of an unprovoked seizure as opposed to recurrent unprovoked seizures (epilepsy), the latter being the primary concern of most patients, families, and clinicians. Of note, a later cohort study found that 6% of children with complex febrile seizures subsequently developed epilepsy.[2]

Question

What is the risk of a subsequent unprovoked seizure in children with febrile seizures?

Answer

In general, there is a 7% overall risk of a subsequent unprovoked seizure, but this risk varies from as low as 2% for simple febrile seizures to almost 50% for febrile seizures with multiple complex features (focality, duration ≥30 minutes, and repeated episodes).

References
1. Tsuboi T, Endo S. Febrile convulsions followed by nonfebrile convulsions. A clinical, electroencephalographic and follow-up study. *Neuropadiatrie.* 1977;8(3):209–223.
2. Verity CM, Golding J. Risk of epilepsy after febrile convulsions: A national cohort study. *BMJ.* 1991; 303(6814):1373–1376.

PRIMARY CARE

71. Long-acting Reversible Contraception in Adolescents
72. Treatment of Acute Otitis Media
73. Childhood Obesity and Cardiovascular Risk
74. Sexually Transmitted Infection Prevalence
75. Cold Medication for Nocturnal Cough in Children
76. Effect of Low-level Lead Exposure on Intellectual
    Impairment
77. Measles, Mumps, and Rubella Vaccination and Autism
78. Risk of Sudden Infant Death Syndrome With Sleeping Factors

CHAPTER 71

LONG-ACTING REVERSIBLE CONTRACEPTION IN ADOLESCENTS

Rachel S. Sagor ■ Elisabeth B. Winterkorn

Provision of No-cost, Long-acting Contraception and Teenage Pregnancy

Secura GM, Madden T, McNicholas C, et al. *N Engl J Med.* 2014;371(14):1316–1323

BACKGROUND

While the US teenage pregnancy rate has declined over the past 2 decades, it remains the highest among developed nations. Long-acting reversible contraceptive (LARC) methods, including intrauterine devices (IUD) and implants are the most effective contraception available. However, lack of information, high cost, and limited access remain barriers to LARC use by adolescents. This study sought to determine whether educating teenage patients about the benefits of contraception and providing them with no-cost access to these agents could reduce the rate of teenage pregnancy.

OBJECTIVES

To determine rates of pregnancy, live birth, and induced abortion in young women educated about and provided with no-cost reversible contraception with an emphasis on LARC.

METHODS

Prospective cohort study in a large metropolitan area in the US from 2007 to 2011.

Patients

1,404 English- or Spanish-speaking females ages 14 to 19 years participating in a larger contraception study. All participants were sexually active or planning to be sexually active with a man within 6 months, willing to switch to a new contraceptive method or not currently using any method, and had no desire to be pregnant within 12 months. Select exclusion criteria: prior hysterectomy or other sterilization procedure.

Intervention

All participants received standardized contraceptive counseling, discussing methods from most to least effective with an emphasis on LARC, and rapid initiation of chosen method at no cost. Outcomes were tracked by telephone for 2 to 3 years. Data were compared to nationally observed rates among all US teens and sexually experienced teens.

Outcomes

Primary outcomes were rates of pregnancy, live birth, and induced abortion. Secondary outcomes were these rates stratified according to age and race, and contraceptive failure rates.

KEY RESULTS

- Study participants had significantly reduced pregnancy rates per 1,000 teens (34 vs. 158.5, 95% CI 25.7–44.1) and birth rates per 1,000 teens (19.4 vs. 94, 95% CI 13.3–27.4) as compared to sexually experienced teens.
- 72% of all participants chose LARC methods, with younger teens preferring implants (50%) and older teens preferring IUDs (42%).
- There were 56 total pregnancies; none occurred with copper IUD or etonogestrel subdermal implant, and only 2 occurred with levonorgestrel IUD (5.1 failures/1,000 teen-years).

STUDY CONCLUSIONS

With the reduction of financial and access barriers to LARC, many adolescents chose this method with associated reduction in pregnancy, birth, and abortion rates as compared to national data.

COMMENTARY

This study showed that informed contraceptive decision making with removal of financial burden is associated with decreased pregnancy rates among teens. Additionally, counseling with emphasis on the safety and success rates of LARC translated into increased interest in these methods compared to observed national rates. Potential limitations of the data include possible underestimation with self-reported pregnancy rates, increased adherence due to regularly scheduled follow-up, and recruitment of a lower-risk cohort due to a parental consent requirement. The Centers for Disease Control and Prevention's Winnable Battle 2015 goal for teen births is a 20% reduction to 30.3 per 1,000 teens; this study emphasizes that much lower rates can be achieved. These results underscore the importance of pediatricians becoming more comfortable recommending and prescribing LARC methods.

Question

Is LARC effective at reducing teen pregnancy?

Answer

Yes, LARC is a safe, desirable, and highly effective way to reduce teen pregnancy.

CHAPTER 72

TREATMENT OF ACUTE OTITIS MEDIA

Jenna M. O'Connell ■ Elisabeth B. Winterkorn

Treatment of Acute Otitis Media in Children Under 2 Years of Age

Hoberman A, Paradise JL, Rockette HE, et al. *N Engl J Med.* 2011;364(2):105–115

BACKGROUND

Approximately 634 per 1,000 children are diagnosed with AOM each year, and although many improve spontaneously, 80% are treated with antibiotics.[1] In 2004, the American Academy of Pediatrics (AAP) endorsed watchful waiting for well-appearing children 6 to 23 months of age with mild disease or an uncertain diagnosis. However, prior studies lacked strict diagnostic criteria for AOM and included children who received suboptimal antibiotic dosing, raising concern about widespread adoption of this strategy.

OBJECTIVES

To determine the impact of antibiotics in resolution of AOM.

METHODS

Double-blind, randomized, placebo-controlled trial at 1 US children's hospital and an affiliated outpatient practice from 2006 to 2009.

Patients

291 patients ages 6 to 23 months with stringently diagnosed AOM confirmed with otoendoscopic pictures (symptom onset <48 hours, symptoms rated by parents ≥3 on the Acute Otitis Media Severity of Symptoms [AOM-SOS] scale, middle ear effusion, and moderate or marked bulging of the tympanic membrane [TM], or slight bulging plus either otalgia or marked TM erythema). Select exclusion criteria: chronic illness, >1 antibiotic dose within 96 hours, receipt of <2 pneumococcal vaccines.

Intervention

Administration of a 10-day course of amoxicillin-clavulanate (90 mg/kg/d amoxicillin divided twice daily) or placebo. Daily phone calls were made until follow-up visit at day 4-5; subsequent visits were at day 10-12 and day 21-25.

Outcomes

Primary outcomes were symptom burden and time to symptom resolution. Secondary outcomes were clinical efficacy, acetaminophen use, adverse events, nasopharyngeal colonization rates, and healthcare resource use.

> ### KEY RESULTS
> * Sustained symptom resolution in treatment group occurred in 20% by day 2, 41% by day 4, and 67% by day 7, as compared to 14%, 36%, and 53% in the placebo group ($p = 0.04$).

- The mean AOM-SOS scores over the first 7 days were lower in the treatment group ($p = 0.02$), with most pronounced effect in children with initial scores >8 (difference of 0.91, 95% CI 0.13–1.68).
- Treatment group was less likely to have clinical failure at the day 4-5 visit (4% vs. 23%, p <0.001) and at the day 10-12 visit (16% vs. 51%, p <0.001).
- There was no significant difference between groups in colonization rates with nonsusceptible *Streptococcus pneumoniae*, doses of acetaminophen administered, or resource use.
- Higher rates of diarrhea (25% vs. 15%, $p = 0.05$) and diaper dermatitis (51% vs. 35%, $p = 0.008$) developed in the treatment group.

STUDY CONCLUSIONS

Children ages 6 to 23 months with AOM treated with 10 days of amoxicillin-clavulanate had improved short-term outcomes as compared to placebo.

COMMENTARY

This study supports the use of antibiotics in decreasing symptom severity and duration in young children with AOM.[1] Limitation was use of amoxicillin-clavulanate as opposed to first-line therapy amoxicillin, though authors stated this was done given prior data showing it was the most effective choice. Based on these data, the AAP guidelines were revised in 2013 to recommend early antibiotic treatment in young children with clear clinical signs of AOM.[2] A watchful waiting approach is still appropriate for children with unilateral and mild disease.

Question

Does treatment with amoxicillin-clavulanate improve outcomes in children 6 to 23 months with acute otitis media?

Answer

Yes, antibiotic treatment shortens symptom duration and decreases clinical failure, with effects most pronounced in patients with more severe presenting disease. Antibiotic side effects underscore the need for use of stringent diagnostic criteria.

References

1. Grijalva CG, Nuorti JP, Griffin MR. Antibiotic prescription rates for acute respiratory tract infections in US ambulatory settings. *JAMA.* 2009;302(7):758–766.
2. Lieberthal AS, Carroll AE, Chonmaitree T, et al. The diagnosis and management of acute otitis media. *Pediatrics.* 2013;131:e964–e999.

CHILDHOOD OBESITY AND CARDIOVASCULAR RISK

CHAPTER 73

Jenna M. O'Connell ■ Elisabeth B. Winterkorn

Childhood Adiposity, Adult Adiposity, and Cardiovascular Risk Factors

Juonala M, Magnussen CG, Berenson GS, et al. *N Engl J Med.* 2011;365(20):1876–1885

BACKGROUND
The prevalence of childhood obesity worldwide has increased in the past several decades particularly in developed countries.[1] Childhood obesity is a known risk factor for persistent obesity and cardiovascular disease (CVD) in adulthood, with associated higher rates of hypertension, dyslipidemia, type 2 diabetes (T2DM), and mortality. It was unknown whether the increased risk of CVD persisted in individuals who were obese as children but became nonobese by adulthood.

OBJECTIVES
To assess whether risk of CVD is lower in overweight or obese children who become nonobese as adults as compared to those who remain obese.

METHODS
Meta-analysis of data from 4 prospective cohort studies (2 US, 1 Australia, and 1 Finland) initiated between 1970 and 1988.

Patients
6,328 children ages 4 to 18 with normal and elevated body mass indices (BMIs) followed for a mean of 23.1 years. Select exclusion criteria: none.

Intervention
Comparison of presence of CVD risk factors related to adiposity status in childhood (age- and sex-adjusted BMI percentiles) and adulthood (BMI ≥25 for overweight, ≥30 obese), comparing normalization of adiposity status vs. the persistence of obesity into adulthood.

Outcomes
Primary outcomes were rates of T2DM, hypertension, dyslipidemia, and high-risk carotid artery intima-media thickness.

KEY RESULTS
- 82.3% of patients who were obese as children remained obese as adults.
- Patients who were obese as children and remained obese as adults had higher rates of T2DM (RR 5.4, 95% CI 3.4–8.5), hypertension (RR 2.7, 95% CI 2.2–3.3), elevated LDL (RR 1.8, 95% CI 1.4–2.3), reduced HDL (RR 2.1, 95% CI 1.8–2.5),

elevated triglycerides (RR 3.0, 95% CI 2.4–3.8), and carotid artery atherosclerosis (RR 1.7, 95% CI 1.4–2.2) than those who were normal weight throughout life.
- Overweight children who had normal BMI as adults had similar risks of all outcomes as individuals with persistently normal BMI (p >0.20 for all comparisons).
- When controlled for adult obesity, associations between childhood obesity and adverse health outcomes were nonsignificant, except hypertension, for which risk was attenuated but remained elevated (RR 1.5, 95% CI 1.1–2.1).

STUDY CONCLUSIONS

Obesity in childhood was associated with an increased rate of CVD risk factors in adulthood, but this returned to baseline for most measures in those who developed a normal BMI by adulthood.

COMMENTARY

This study confirmed that childhood obesity is a risk factor for several CVD risk factors in adulthood; however, it found that normalization of BMI by adulthood mitigates this risk. Further research is needed to determine the long-term impact of childhood obesity on rates of cardiovascular events and mortality. Of note, they studied a predominantly Caucasian population which is not generalizable to other populations such as blacks or Hispanics. Though limited by its observational nature, this study should encourage pediatricians to counsel overweight children about a healthy diet and exercise with the goal of normalizing BMI by adulthood. It also supports efforts to promote and maintain healthy lifestyles for all children.

Question

In overweight and obese children, is normalization of BMI by adulthood protective against development of cardiovascular risk factors?

Answer

Yes, patients who are overweight or obese as children but have normal BMIs as adults have similar rates of nearly all cardiovascular risk factors to those who are nonobese throughout their life.

Reference

1. Wang Y, Lobstein T. Worldwide trends in childhood overweight and obesity. *Int J Pediatr Obes.* 2006;1:11–25.

SEXUALLY TRANSMITTED INFECTION PREVALENCE

CHAPTER 74

Jenna M. O'Connell ■ Elisabeth B. Winterkorn

Prevalence of Sexually Transmitted Infections Among Female Adolescents Aged 14 to 19 in the United States

Forhan SE, Gottlieb SL, Sternberg MR, et al. *Pediatrics.* 2009;124(6):1505–1512

BACKGROUND

Adolescence is a common time for initiation of sexual activity and first exposure to sexually transmitted infections (STI), with risks of pelvic inflammatory disease, infertility, and cervical cancer. Although community-based studies demonstrated high rates of STIs in specific adolescent populations, no large-scale data existed. This study aimed to gather data to inform prevention efforts.

OBJECTIVES

To measure prevalence of STIs in adolescent females in a representative US sample.

METHODS

Prospective, observational study using data from the National Health and Nutrition Examination Survey (NHANES), a large survey of the US population on health-related issues, from 2003 to 2004.

Patients

838 females ages 14 to 19. Select exclusion criteria: institutionalized individuals.

Intervention

Determination of STI prevalence (as detected in urine, serum, and vaginal swab specimens) in relation to age and sexual history, assessed through standard interview, physical examination, and sexual history.

Outcomes

Primary outcome was prevalence of ≥1 of 5 STIs: *Neisseria gonorrhoeae, Chlamydia trachomatis* (chlamydia), *Trichomonas vaginalis,* herpes simplex virus type 2 (HSV2), and human papillomavirus (HPV), focusing on 23 high-risk types, type 6, or 11 (HR/6/11). Secondary outcome was prevalence of individual STIs.

KEY RESULTS
- Overall prevalence of any STI was 24.1% (95% CI 18.4–30.9).
- The most prevalent STIs were HPV HR/6/11 (18.3%, 95% CI 13.5–24.8) and chlamydia (3.9%, 95% CI 2.2–6.9).
- Of all individuals with an STI, 15.8% had >1 STI (95% CI 11.2–21.8).

- Prevalence of STI in those with <1-year duration of sexual activity was 25.6% (95% CI 16.3–37.8) and in those with 1 partner was 19.7% (95% CI 12.3–29.9). Notably, prevalence in those reporting 0 lifetime partners was 6.6% (95% CI 2.7–15).
- On multivariate analysis, non-Hispanic black participants had increased odds of having ≥1 STI when compared to non-Hispanic whites (adjusted OR 3.6, 95% CI 1.9–6.8).

STUDY CONCLUSIONS

The prevalence of STIs in adolescent females was high, supporting the need for early and comprehensive sex education, universal HPV vaccination in preadolescence, and chlamydia screening for all sexually active females.

COMMENTARY

This was the first publication of the national prevalence of STIs among adolescent females, showing high prevalence, even in girls who reported minimal or no prior sexual activity. Based on this and other studies, a 2014 American Academy of Pediatrics Policy Statement recommended chlamydia screening for all sexually active female adolescents.[1] Although limited by self-reported data and exclusion of STIs such as HIV and syphilis (only screened for in 18 and 19 year olds), these data should encourage pediatricians to initiate preventative counseling, HPV vaccination, and universal screening during adolescence. Unfortunately, in 2013, only 37.6% of girls aged 13 to 17 had completed the HPV vaccine series, with fewer black females having received all 3 doses when compared to whites and Hispanics.[2] The racial disparity found in these studies underscores the need for ongoing efforts to ensure that all subpopulations receive optimal education and screening.

Question

How prevalent are the most common STIs in adolescent females in the US?

Answer

Nearly 1 out of 4 female adolescents have at least 1 STI, with HPV accounting for the majority. The prevalence was high even in those who reported recent onset of sexual activity or only having few sexual partners.

References

1. Committee on Adolescence; Society for Adolescent Health and Medicine. Screening for nonviral sexually transmitted infections in adolescents and young adults. *Pediatrics.* 2014;134(1):e302–e311.
2. Centers for Disease Control and Prevention. Teen vaccination coverage. 2013 national immunization survey-teen (nis-teen). Available at: http://www.cdc.gov/vaccines/who/teens/vaccination-coverage.html. Modified on July 24, 2014. Accessed on July 9, 2015.

CHAPTER 75

COLD MEDICATION FOR NOCTURNAL COUGH IN CHILDREN

Jenna M. O'Connell ■ Elisabeth B. Winterkorn

Effect of Dextromethorphan, Diphenhydramine, and Placebo on Nocturnal Cough and Sleep Quality for Coughing Children and Their Parents

Paul IM, Yoder KE, Crowell KR, et al. *Pediatrics.* 2004;114(1):e85–e90

BACKGROUND

Cough is one of the most bothersome symptoms for children with upper respiratory tract infections (URI), and leads to more ambulatory visits than any other symptom.[1] Parents and physicians often used over-the-counter (OTC) treatments to alleviate these symptoms, despite lack of evidence showing a clear benefit and documented risk of side effects. This study sought to assess prospectively whether common remedies were beneficial.

OBJECTIVES

To determine whether dextromethorphan (DM) or diphenhydramine (DPH) improves nocturnal cough in children with acute cough from URI as compared to placebo.

METHODS

Double-blind, randomized, placebo-controlled trial in 2 US pediatric outpatient practices from 2002 to 2003.

Patients

100 patients ages 2 to 16 years with cough attributable to URI (rhinorrhea and cough for ≤7 days). Select exclusion criteria: treatment ≤24 hours with DM or DPH, evidence of a treatable illness causing cough (including pneumonia or croup), asthma, chronic lung disease, or allergic rhinitis.

Intervention

Subjects were randomly assigned to receive weight-based doses of DM, DPH, or placebo (simple syrup) 30 minutes before bed. Parental assessments of cough and sleep difficulty were assessed using a 7-point Likert scale on day of presentation and day following intervention by telephone.

Outcomes

Primary outcome was frequency of cough. Secondary outcomes were cough severity, sleep quality for both child and parent, and degree of distress caused by cough for the child and parent.

KEY RESULTS

- Patients in placebo, DM, and DPH groups showed improvement in all outcomes on night 2 with mean combined symptom score reduction from 19.83 to 8.93 (95% CI for reduction 9.38–12.42).

- There were no significant differences among treatment groups and placebo in outcomes ($p = 0.62$).
- Drowsiness occurred in 3 children in the DPH group, as compared to 0 in the other groups ($p = 0.07$).
- Insomnia occurred in 3 children in the DM group, as compared to 0 in the other groups ($p = 0.07$).

STUDY CONCLUSIONS

DM and DPH performed no better than placebo in relieving nocturnal cough or improving sleep quality for children with URIs or for parents.

COMMENTARY

Parents in all 3 groups reported improvement in symptoms on the night after medication administration, which may represent placebo effect or the natural course of illness. Of concern, there was a trend toward increased side effects with DM and DPH, and other studies have documented risk of overdose associated with both in children.[2] There may be confounding, as patients concomitantly treated with acetaminophen or ibuprofen were not excluded, and it was slightly underpowered. Nonetheless, based on this and similar studies demonstrating unfavorable risk–benefit profiles, OTC cold medications for children under age 4 were withdrawn from the market in 2007. The American Academy of Pediatrics now recommends honey as a safe and low-cost alternative that can be helpful in improving cough in children >1 year of age.[3]

Question

Do OTC cold medications improve nocturnal cough in children with upper respiratory infections?

Answer

No, neither DM nor DPH performs better than placebo in improving cough or sleep for children or their parents, and should be avoided in children under age 4.

References

1. Cherry DK, Woodwell DA. National ambulatory medical care survey: 2000 summary. *Adv Data*. 2002; (328):1–32.
2. Centers for Disease Control and Prevention (CDC). Infant deaths associated with cough and cold medications–two states, 2005. *MMWR Morb Mortal Wkly Rep.* 2007;56(1):1–4.
3. American Academy of Pediatrics. Coughs and colds: Medicines or home remedies? Available at: https://www.healthychildren.org/English/health-issues/conditions/chest-lungs/Pages/Coughs-and-Colds-Medicines-or-Home-Remedies.aspx. Modified on May 5, 2015. Accessed on July 8, 2015.

CHAPTER 76

EFFECT OF LOW-LEVEL LEAD EXPOSURE ON INTELLECTUAL IMPAIRMENT

Jenna M. O'Connell ■ Elisabeth B. Winterkorn

Intellectual Impairment in Children With Blood Lead Concentrations Below 10 Micrograms Per Deciliter

Canfield RL, Henderson CR Jr, Cory-Slechta DA, et al. *N Engl J Med.* 2003;348(16): 1517–1526

BACKGROUND

Numerous studies have demonstrated neurotoxic effects of lead levels above 10 mcg/dL, particularly in young children. Adverse outcomes include impairment in intellectual functioning and social-behavioral conduct. The Centers for Disease Control and Prevention (CDC) and World Health Organization (WHO) had previously designated 10 mcg/dL as a level of concern; however, it remained unclear whether cognitive deficits could occur in children with lower levels.

OBJECTIVES

To observe whether impaired performance on intelligence testing occurs at blood lead concentrations <10 mcg/dL.

METHODS

Prospective cohort study of children born in 1 US city between 1994 and 1995.

Patients

172 children ages 24 to 30 months. Select exclusion criteria: prematurity, low birth weight, trisomy 21, speech or hearing abnormalities.

Intervention

Blood lead levels measured 7 times from 6 to 60 months of age compared with rates of intellectual impairment on the Stanford–Binet Intelligence Scale (IQ), administered at ages 3 and 5 years.

Outcomes

Primary outcomes were 4 measures of degree of lead exposure (lifetime average, peak, random on the day of cognitive testing, and average in infancy) and intellectual impairment.

KEY RESULTS

- After adjustment for covariates (including sex, birth weight, iron status, maternal IQ, tobacco exposure), IQ scores were inversely associated with average lifetime blood lead levels ($p = 0.004$).
- For every increase in the lifetime average blood lead level of 1 mcg/dL, IQ score fell by 0.46 points (95% CI −0.76 to −0.15).

- Even in children whose blood lead level was persistently <10 mcg/dL, each incremental elevation in lifetime average blood level of 1 mcg/dL resulted in a 1.37 point decrease in IQ level (95% CI −2.56 to −0.17).
- Lifetime average concentrations that were elevated but <10 mcg/dL led to a decline of 7.4 IQ points, whereas from 10 to 30 mcg/dL the subsequent loss was more gradual, estimated at only 2.5 points.

STUDY CONCLUSIONS
Blood lead levels early in childhood were inversely and significantly associated with IQ scores at 3 and 5 years of age, with the steepest decline in IQ due to initial lead exposures seen at levels 2 to 10 mcg/dL.

COMMENTARY

Although observational, this study dramatically showed that even low-level exposure negatively affects IQ later in childhood. Subsequently, another observational study also revealed an association between low-level lead exposure and neurodevelopmental outcomes,[1] prompting the CDC to revise the definition for elevated blood lead level to <5 mcg/dL, a reference value based on the 97.5th percentile of the distribution among children 1 to 5 years old.[2] Current guidelines recommend focus on primary prevention, family education, and environmental assessments to identify sources of lead exposure given the potentially irreversible neurodevelopmental effects and absence of treatments for low-level exposure. Of note, lower income, nonwhite race, lower level of maternal education, and low maternal IQ were correlated with higher lead levels, highlighting particular populations to target with prevention efforts.

Question
Is low-level lead exposure associated with intellectual impairment?

Answer
Yes, elevated blood lead levels even when <10 mcg/dL are significantly associated with lower intelligence quotients in young children, emphasizing the importance of primary prevention of exposure.

References
1. Téllez-Rojo MM, Bellinger DC, Arroyo-Quiroz C, et al. Longitudinal associations between blood lead concentrations lower than 10 microg/dL and neurobehavioral development in environmentally exposed children in Mexico City. *Pediatrics.* 2006;118(2):e323–e330.
2. Centers for Disease Control and Prevention (CDC). CDC response to advisory committee on childhood lead poisoning prevention recommendations in "low level lead exposure harms children: A renewed call of primary prevention." Available at: http://www.cdc.gov/nceh/lead/ACCLPP/CDC_Response_Lead_Exposure_Recs.pdf. Modified on June 7, 2012. Accessed on July 9, 2015.

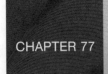

MEASLES, MUMPS, AND RUBELLA VACCINATION AND AUTISM

CHAPTER 77

Eliza G. Stensland ■ Elisabeth B. Winterkorn

A Population-based Study of Measles, Mumps, and Rubella Vaccination and Autism

Madsen KM, Hviid A, Vestergaard M, et al. *N Engl J Med.* 2002;347(19):1477–1482

BACKGROUND
The alleged link between the measles, mumps, and rubella (MMR) vaccine and autism made by Wakefield et al.[1] engendered significant fear and mistrust of potential side effects of vaccination, leading to increased immunization refusal. Though the original article was retracted due to the use of fraudulent data, the rising incidence of autism and related diagnoses has fueled persistent interest in the suggested correlation. Earlier studies looking at the relationship were either case series or cross sectional; this was the first study assessing the association between MMR vaccine and autism that was adequately powered.

OBJECTIVES
To assess the RR of MMR vaccination and diagnosis of autism or autism spectrum disorder (ASD).

METHODS
Retrospective cohort study reviewing 6 national registries of all children born in Denmark from 1991 to 1998.

Patients
537,303 children born during the specified time frame. Select exclusion criteria: genetic conditions associated with an increased risk of ASD (tuberous sclerosis, congenital rubella, fragile X, and Angelman syndrome), loss to follow-up.

Intervention
MMR vaccine administration by 15 months of age was compared to no administration. The Danish Psychiatric Central Register, which contains information on all psychiatric diagnoses, provided autism diagnostic data.

Outcomes
Primary outcome was diagnosis of autism or ASD by a child psychiatrist prior to the study's conclusion using the Diagnostic and Statistical Manual-IV diagnostic criteria.

KEY RESULTS
- 440,655 received MMR vaccine by age 15 months; 96,648 children did not. 98.5% of all children were vaccinated before age 3 with a mean age of 17 months at time of vaccination.

- 316 children were diagnosed with autism and 422 with ASD.
- After adjusting for age, calendar period, sex, birth weight, gestational age, socio-economic status, and maternal education, there was no significant difference in incidence of autism or ASD in vaccinated children compared to unvaccinated children; RR 0.92 (95% CI 0.68–1.24) for autism and RR 0.83 (95% CI 0.65–1.07) for ASD, respectively.
- There were no associations between development of an autistic disorder and age at vaccination ($p = 0.23$), time since vaccination ($p = 0.42$), or month of vaccination ($p = 0.06$).

STUDY CONCLUSIONS

MMR vaccination was not associated with an increased risk of autism or ASD, nor was there a temporal association between vaccination and autism/ASD diagnosis.

COMMENTARY

This was the first large population-level study adequately powered to examine the possible association between the MMR vaccination and a diagnosis of ASD while controlling for possible confounders. It showed no clustering of diagnosis around vaccination and provided strong arguments against a causal relationship, which had been noted earlier in the literature.[1] Importantly, that association has never been reproduced and the original article has since been retracted.[2] Even though it has been over a decade since this article's publication, vaccination remains a highly contentious issue. Therefore, papers such as this continue to be highly important both on a policy level and on an individual level as reassurance for concerned parents.

Question

Is the MMR vaccine associated with an increased risk of autism or ASD?

Answer

No, this large retrospective cohort of children showed no increased risk of being diagnosed with autism or ASD after having been vaccinated with the MMR vaccine.

References

1. Wakefield AJ, Murch SH, Anthony A, et al. Ileal-lymphoid-nodular hyperplasia, non-specific colitis, and pervasive developmental disorder in children. *Lancet.* 1998;351(9103):637–641.
2. Retraction–Ileal-lymphoid-nodular hyperplasia, non-specific colitis, and pervasive developmental disorder in children. *Lancet.* 2010;375(9713):445.

RISK OF SUDDEN INFANT DEATH SYNDROME WITH SLEEPING FACTORS

Eliza G. Stensland ■ Elisabeth B. Winterkorn

Interaction Between Bedding and Sleeping Position in the Sudden Infant Death Syndrome: A Population Based Case-Control Study

Fleming PJ, Gilbert R, Azaz Y, et al. *BMJ*. 1990;301(6743):85–89

BACKGROUND
Through the early 1990s, the rate of sudden infant death syndrome (SIDS), now known as sudden unexpected infant death (SUID), was 1.3:1,000 births in the United States.[1] Contemporaneous studies suggested a possible role of thermal stress or prone positioning during sleep as a causative factor in SIDS.

OBJECTIVES
To determine the relationship of sleep position and bedding on incidence of SIDS.

METHODS
Case-control study in the United Kingdom from 1987 to 1989.

Patients
67 index SIDS cases age ≤1 year who died of SIDS and 144 age-matched controls. Select exclusion criteria: identified cause of death.

Intervention
Prevalence of sleep position, bedding, infant temperature, and environmental temperature in cases were compared to controls. For each death, 2 infants living in the same neighborhood and of similar age were identified. Families of the cases and controls were interviewed about infants' medical and social histories; detailed information about their sleep position, clothing, and bedding was also obtained. Using previously published data on thermal resistance of specific materials, total thermal resistance of bedding material (indicated by the tog value) was calculated.

Outcomes
Primary outcome was infant death.

KEY RESULTS
- 138 of 201 infants (69%) slept prone.
- Infants who died from SIDS were significantly more likely to have been sleeping prone (RR 8.8, 95% CI 7–11) and/or heavily wrapped (RR 1.14 per tog above 8 tog, 95% CI 1.03–1.28). Infants who died from SIDS were also more likely to have used in-home heating at night (RR 2.7, 95% CI 1.4–5.2).

- The weights of the infants who died were statistically lower than the controls (p <0.01).
- When stratified by age, there were differences in thermal resistance (p <0.01) and prone positioning (p <0.001) between the cases and controls in those ≥70 days old. In those <70 days old, only the difference in prone position was statistically significant (RR 4.15, 95% CI 1.32–13.04).

STUDY CONCLUSIONS

Prone sleeping position and excess heating (either from bedding or ambient temperature) were independently associated with increased risk of SIDS, especially in infants ≥70 days.

COMMENTARY

This study was fundamental in informing the current American Academy of Pediatrics recommendation that infants sleep in a supine position and in an empty crib, without excess bundling or blankets. It continues to have a lasting impact on educational campaigns such as "Back-to-Sleep" and the rate of SUID declined to 0.39 in 1,000 births in 2013. It is important to note that the recommended interventions are low cost and low risk, and easily understood by parents and physicians. Concerns have arisen about other practices, such as cosleeping, and recent studies continue to elucidate which features of unsafe sleeping environments play the largest role.[2]

Question

Are there identifiable risk factors that increase the risk of SUID?

Answer

Yes, this study demonstrated an increased risk of SUID in infants who slept in a prone position and were more heavily wrapped during sleep. This was most pronounced in infants ≥70 days old.

References

1. Centers for Disease Control and Prevention, National Center for Chronic Disease Prevention and Health Promotion. "Sudden unexpected infant death and sudden infant death syndrome." Available at: www.cdc.gov/sids/data.htm. Accessed on July 20, 2015.
2. Colvin JD, Collie-Akers V, Schunn C, et al. Sleep environment risks for younger and older infants. *Pediatrics.* 2014;134(2):e406–e412.

PSYCHIATRY/ DEVELOPMENT

79. Medications Versus Cognitive Behavioral Therapy
 in the Treatment of Depression
80. Medication Versus Behavioral Treatment in Attention
 Deficit Hyperactivity Disorder
81. Childhood Psychosocial Stress and Adult Disease
82. Effect of Early Developmental Intervention in
 Preterm Infants
83. Behavioral Intervention for Autism

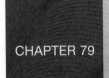

MEDICATIONS VERSUS COGNITIVE BEHAVIORAL THERAPY IN THE TREATMENT OF DEPRESSION

CHAPTER 79

Rachel S. Sagor ■ Elizabeth Pinsky

Fluoxetine, Cognitive-Behavioral Therapy, and Their Combination for Adolescents With Depression: Treatment for Adolescents With Depression Study (TADS) Randomized Controlled Trial

March J, Silva S, Petrycki S, et al. *JAMA.* 2004;292(7):807–820

BACKGROUND

Major depressive disorder (MDD) has a prevalence of approximately 9% among 12 to 17 year olds, and is associated with significant comorbidities including suicidality, long-term disease persistence, and adult psychosocial impairment.[1] Standard therapy for MDD in adolescents has included selective serotonin reuptake inhibitors (SSRI) and cognitive-behavioral therapy (CBT). Adult data suggested that combination therapy led to greater symptom improvement over monotherapy; however, no such studies existed among the adolescent population.

OBJECTIVES

To compare the effectiveness of placebo vs. SSRI therapy and CBT both alone and in combination for treatment of adolescent depression.

METHODS

Randomized controlled trial at 13 US clinics from 2000 to 2003.

Patients

439 patients ages 12 to 17 years with Diagnostic and Statistical Manual of Mental Disorders IV (DSM-IV) diagnosis of MDD, Children's Depression Rating Scale-Revised (CDRS-R) score >45, and depressive mood in 2 of 3 contexts (home, school, among peers) for >6 weeks. Select exclusion criteria: current psychiatric medication or therapy, psychiatric hospitalization <3 months prior, significant suicide or homicide risk.

Intervention

12 weeks of SSRI alone (fluoxetine 10 to 40 mg/d with 6 × 20–30 minute pharmacotherapy visits), CBT alone (15 × 50–60 minute sessions), CBT + SSRI, or placebo. SSRI alone and placebo were double-blinded.

Outcomes

Primary outcomes were CDRS-R score and Clinical Global Impression (CGI) score at baseline, 6, and 12 weeks. Secondary outcomes included suicidality and adverse events.

KEY RESULTS

- SSRI + CBT was the superior treatment for depression with an improvement in CGI score of 71.0% (95% CI 62–80) compared to SSRI (60.6%, 95% CI 51–70), CBT (43.2%, 95% CI 34–52), or placebo (34.8%, 95% CI 26–44).
- At baseline, patients had a rate of suicidal thinking of 29%. All 4 treatment groups showed a significant reduction, with the greatest response in the SSRI + CBT group ($p = 0.02$). Effect sizes suggested that CBT had a small but protective effect on suicidal ideation.
- No significant difference in suicide-related events among any group was noted.

STUDY CONCLUSIONS

For adolescents with MDD, a combination of CBT + SSRI offered superior improvement in depression score and greatest protection against suicidality.

COMMENTARY

This pivotal study demonstrated that combination therapy for MDD was superior to monotherapy in adolescents. Given concerns raised by the Food and Drug Administration "black box" warning on increased suicidality associated with adolescent SSRI use, this study reassured providers as all groups had reductions in suicidal ideation, with CBT demonstrating a small but protective effect. Longer-term TADS analyses have since shown that all treatment arms have equivalent outcomes at 36 weeks, suggesting overall that combined treatment results in faster remission, and that CBT enhances safety of medications.[2] These studies offer providers the clearest data yet to help guide parents and adolescents in shared decision making around treatment of depression.

Question

What is the most efficacious and safe treatment regimen for an adolescent with MDD?

Answer

Combination therapy with an SSRI and CBT is shown to have the greatest improvement in symptoms and suicidality.

References

1. Substance Abuse and Mental Health Services Administration. *Results From the 2012 National Survey on Drug Use and Health: Mental Health Findings,* NSDUH Series H-47, HHS Publication No. (SMA) 13–4805. Rockville, MD: Substance Abuse and Mental Health Services Administration; 2013.
2. March JS, Silva S, Petrycki S. The Treatment for Adolescents With Depression Study (TADS): Long-term effectiveness and safety outcomes. *Arch Gen Psychiatry.* 2007;64(10):1132–1143.

MEDICATION VERSUS BEHAVIORAL TREATMENT IN ATTENTION DEFICIT HYPERACTIVITY DISORDER

CHAPTER 80

Rachel S. Sagor ■ Elizabeth Pinsky

A 14-Month Randomized Clinical Trial of Treatment Strategies for Attention-Deficit/ Hyperactivity Disorder. The MTA Cooperative Group. Multimodal Treatment Study of Children With ADHD

Arch Gen Psychiatry. 1999;56(12):1073–1086

BACKGROUND

Attention deficit hyperactivity disorder (ADHD), the most common psychiatric illness among children, has significant effects on social, familial, and academic functioning. Management typically includes medications, behavioral treatment, or a combination of these. Despite short-term data regarding efficacy of these 2 modalities, prior to this study there were no long-term (>4 months) studies comparing these time-intensive interventions.

OBJECTIVES

To compare long-term outcomes of different treatment modalities in the management of ADHD.

METHODS

Randomized controlled trial at 6 US sites from 1994 to 1998.

Patients

579 children ages 7 to 9 years who met Diagnostic and Statistical Manual of Mental Disorders IV (DSM-IV) criteria for ADHD, combined type. Select exclusion criteria: inability to participate in interventions, treatment requirements beyond study ability.

Intervention

Participants were randomized to one of four 14-month long treatments: intensive medication management (monthly 30-minute medication visits); intensive behavioral treatment (parent training, child-focused treatment, and school-based interventions); combination intensive management (all components of intensive medication management and behavioral treatment); or standard community care (formal initial evaluation and subsequent care at provider's discretion). Side effects were monitored monthly using parent rating scales.

Outcomes

Primary outcomes included ADHD symptoms, aggression, internalizing symptoms, social skills, and parent–child relations. Secondary outcomes included adverse medication effects.

KEY RESULTS

- Intensive medication management and combination management were superior to intensive behavioral treatment or standard community care in reducing ADHD symptoms ($p \leq 0.002$), despite the fact that 2/3 of children in the standard community care group received medications.
- All groups showed reductions in symptoms of ADHD, aggression, and internalizing.
- When compared to intensive behavioral management or standard community care, combination management significantly reduced non-ADHD symptoms, including aggressive and internalizing symptoms ($p \leq 0.003$), and significantly improved social skills ($p \leq 0.003$), parent–child relations ($p \leq 0.004$), and reading achievement ($p \leq 0.001$).
- Standard community care patients received a lower total daily dose of ADHD medications (22.6 mg) compared to medication management subjects (37.7 mg) and combined treatment subjects (31.2 mg).
- 88% reported no medication adverse effects.

STUDY CONCLUSIONS

Intensive medication management was superior to behavioral management alone or standard community care for ADHD. Combination treatment offered extra benefits beyond treatment of core ADHD symptoms.

COMMENTARY

This study highlights the importance of pharmacologic and behavioral management of ADHD, while also emphasizing that vigilant and robust medication management is paramount. Medication choice, appropriate dose titration, and to a modest extent, intensive behavioral treatment, can lead to significant symptom reduction. Of note, while standard community care used similar modalities and reduced ADHD symptoms, its inferiority was presumably attributable to less intensive pharmacologic interventions. Given that most pediatric patients with ADHD are cared by community providers, continued training in best management strategies must be accessible and promoted. While this was a long-term study, it did not address participant outcomes after their intensive interventions were completed. Subsequently, a prospective follow-up study showed that at 6 to 8 years, prognosis was based largely on early ADHD symptoms rather than specific treatment groups.[1] Together, these studies support assertive medication management for children and indicate that ongoing care and innovative treatments are essential well into adolescence.

Question

What treatment modalities result in the best outcomes and symptom management for children with ADHD?

Answer

Intensive medication management is paramount in the treatment of ADHD symptoms. Behavioral treatment offers modest additional benefits in non-core ADHD symptoms and yields positive functioning outcomes.

Reference

1. Molina BS, Hinshaw SP, Swanson JM, et al. The MTA at 8 Years: Prospective follow-up of children treated for combined type ADHD in a multisite study. *J Am Acad Child Adolesc Psychiatry.* 2009;48(5): 484–500.

CHILDHOOD PSYCHOSOCIAL STRESS AND ADULT DISEASE

CHAPTER 81

Rachel S. Sagor ■ Elizabeth Pinsky

Relationship of Childhood Abuse and Household Dysfunction to Many of the Leading Causes of Death in Adults. The Adverse Childhood Experiences (ACE) Study

Felitti VJ, Anda RF, Nordenberg D, et al. *Am J Prev Med.* 1998;14(4):245–258

BACKGROUND
Leading causes of death among adults have been well studied and are understood to be partly related to both health behaviors and lifestyle factors. Adverse childhood experiences (ACE), particularly abuse, are known to have long-term consequences; however, there had been no previous analysis of ACEs and their contribution to adult behaviors, lifestyle decisions, or disease prevalence. This study sought to understand the role ACEs play in long-term health outcomes.

OBJECTIVES
To measure the relationship between childhood exposure to adverse events and adult household dysfunction, health-risk behaviors, and disease.

METHODS
Retrospective cross-sectional study in a large US urban primary care clinic from 1995 to 1996.

Patients
9,508 adults ages 19 to 92 years. Select exclusion criteria: incomplete questionnaires.

Intervention
All patients underwent a standard medical evaluation including history, physical examination, and laboratory testing. Subsequently they received the ACE study questionnaire. 1 point was attributed for each exposure within 7 categories: childhood abuse (psychological, physical, and sexual) and household dysfunction (substance use, mental illness, mother treated violently, and family member imprisoned).

Outcomes
Primary outcomes were categorized as presence of health-risk factors including smoking, severe obesity, physical inactivity, depressed mood, suicide attempts, alcoholism, drug use, ≥50 lifetime sexual partners, history of sexually transmitted infection (STI) as well as disease conditions including ischemic heart disease, cancer, stroke, chronic bronchitis, emphysema, diabetes, hepatitis, and skeletal fractures.

KEY RESULTS

- 52% of respondents experienced ≥1 ACE, while 6.2% experienced ≥4 ACEs.
- Respondents with ≥4 ACEs compared to those with none had increased risk of suicide attempt (OR 12.2, 95% CI 8.5–17.5), injected drug use (OR 10.3, 95% CI 4.9–21.4), self-identification as alcoholic (OR 7.4, 95% CI 5.4–10.2), and smoking (OR 2.2, 95% CI 1.7–2.9).
- Only 14% of respondents with ≥4 ACEs were without any health-risk factors as compared with 56% of respondents with none.
- Respondents with ≥4 ACEs were at increased risk for numerous disease conditions compared to those with none (OR range 1.6–3.9). There was a dose–response relationship between ACEs and number of health-risk factors and diseases ($p < 0.001$).

STUDY CONCLUSIONS

Higher numbers of ACEs were correlated with increased health-risk factors and disease in adulthood.

COMMENTARY

While it has long been supported that prevention of childhood abuse and exposure to household dysfunction is paramount for pediatric development, this study underscored that long-term health outcomes in adulthood are also profoundly affected by ACEs. The significant contribution to adult morbidity and mortality, and therefore to associated healthcare costs, supports the importance of early initiation of targeted programs and interventions in primary care offices, schools, and homes. These data have been pivotal in the introduction of programs such as "Healthy Steps" which adds developmental specialist visits to routine well childcare during the first 3 years of life. The program has expanded from California to a total of 15 states, representing an approach to mediating childhood risks with potentially profound and far-reaching impacts on adult health.

Question

Is abuse and household dysfunction in childhood associated with worsened health outcomes as an adult?

Answer

Yes, there are significant long-term health risks to those exposed to ACEs, emphasizing the importance of early intervention and prevention of these events.

CHAPTER 82

EFFECT OF EARLY DEVELOPMENTAL INTERVENTION IN PRETERM INFANTS

Lila Worden ■ Elizabeth Pinsky

Enhancing the Outcomes of Low-Birth-Weight, Premature Infants: A Multisite, Randomized Trial. The Infant Health and Development Program
JAMA. 1990;263(22):3035–3042

BACKGROUND

Advancements in neonatal intensive care increased the survival of preterm and low-birth-weight (LBW) infants; however, these infants remained at increased risk of intellectual and learning disabilities, behavioral problems, and medical complications as compared to normal birth weight peers. With the expansion of the Individuals with Disabilities Education Act in 1987, developmentally at-risk infants were newly eligible for early intervention (EI) programs. Previous research on EI programs in LBW populations was limited to small, short-term studies.

OBJECTIVES

To assess the efficacy of comprehensive EI on improving developmental outcomes and physical health of preterm LBW infants.

METHODS

Randomized controlled trial in 8 US centers from 1985 to 1988.

Patients

985 infants followed from birth to 36 months who were born <37 weeks' gestational age (GA) with birth weight ≤2,500 g. Select exclusion criteria: serious health impairment precluding participation.

Intervention

A program that included home visits every 1 to 2 weeks, child care at a child development center from 12 to 36 months of age, parent group meetings, and pediatric follow-up from hospital discharge through 36 months corrected age was compared to standard pediatric preventive care for former preterm infants.

Outcomes

Primary outcomes were differences in cognitive development (measured by the Stanford–Binet Intelligence Scale), behavioral problems (measured by the Child Behavior Checklist), and health status (multiple measures encompassing morbidity, functional status, and maternal perception of health) stratified by heavier (2,001 to 2,500 g) and lighter (≤2,000 g) birth weight.

KEY RESULTS
- Children in the control group were more likely than those receiving EI to have intellectual disability with IQ <70 (OR 2.7, 95% CI 1.6–4.8).
- Heavier LBW infants had more cognitive gain from EI than lighter LBW infants (13 IQ points vs. 7 IQ points, $p = 0.014$).
- Adjusted OR for behavior problems was 1.8 times greater in the control group (95% CI 1.2–2.9). The intervention effect size on behavioral outcomes was lower for infants of college-educated mothers ($p = 0.009$).
- There were no differences in serious morbidity in either group. Lighter LBW infants had greater number of minor illnesses over 3 years (8 vs. 7, p <0.001).

STUDY CONCLUSIONS
Preterm LBW infants who received EI had higher IQs and fewer behavioral problems as compared to controls, with greatest improvement seen in heavier LBW infants and those from families with lower maternal education level.

COMMENTARY
This landmark study demonstrated that comprehensive EI yielded long-term improvements for LBW infants. The study was notable for its strong prospective design, high retention rate (93%), and diverse geographic and demographic populations. Referral of premature infants to EI programs has therefore been the standard of care since the mid-1990s. Since this initial study, it has been shown that at 5 years of age, lighter LBW infants had no sustained effects of EI but heavier LBW infants had continued improvement in IQ and behavior through 18 years of age.[1] While subsequent analyses have shown full-time attendance at child care centers has the most robust effect on long-term development, this level of comprehensive services is often excluded from state-run EI programs and remains underfunded on a national level.

Question
Is intensive EI effective for LBW, preterm infants?

Answer
Yes, intensive EI improves cognitive development and behavior of LBW preterm infants, especially those who are born >2,000 g.

Reference
1. McCormick MC, Brooks-Gunn J, Buka SL, et al. Early intervention in low birth weight premature infants: Results at 18 years of age for the Infant Health and Development Program. *Pediatrics.* 2006;117(3): 771–780.

CHAPTER 83

BEHAVIORAL INTERVENTION FOR AUTISM

Rachel S. Sagor ■ Elizabeth Pinsky

Behavioral Treatment and Normal Educational and Intellectual Functioning in Young Autistic Children

Lovaas OI. *J Consult Clin Psychol.* 1987;55(1):3–9

BACKGROUND

Autism, now reclassified as autism spectrum disorder (ASD), is a pediatric neurodevelopmental disorder characterized by functional deficits in social communication and interaction across multiple contexts. It can lead to significant emotional hardships for families and be financially burdensome on the public health system when left untreated. In the late 1970s, the prognosis for children with autism was poor, as available medical and psychodynamic therapies were ineffective. Favorable anecdotal data on the use of behavioral-targeted therapy had begun to emerge, but no trial had yet tested this promising intervention.

OBJECTIVES

To evaluate the effectiveness of early, intensive behavior modification on intellectual and educational functioning in young children with autism.

METHODS

Nonrandomized controlled trial at a single US center from 1970 to 1986.

Patients

38 children diagnosed with autism according to The Diagnostic and Statistical Manual of Mental Disorders III (DSM-III) criteria, <40 months of age (if mute) or <46 months of age (if echolalic). Select exclusion criteria: mental age of <11 months at 30 months of age.

Intervention

Children were placed in 1 of 2 treatment groups for ≥2 years with preference given to intensive treatment unless staffing was unavailable. The intensive-treatment (experimental) group included 40+ hours of 1:1 treatment with trained student therapists in the home, school, and community as well as caregiver training. The control group included 10 hours of 1:1 treatment. Best efforts were made to continue intensive treatments for the study participants past the 2-year mark.

Outcomes

Primary outcomes included educational placement and intelligence quotient (IQ).

KEY RESULTS

- Pretreatment, the experimental and control groups' chronologic ages were 32 and 35.3 months with mental ages of 18.8 and 17.1 months, respectively.
- At follow-up, experimental group had significantly higher IQ than the control group (83.3 vs. 52.3, p <0.01).
- Only 10% of treatment group had follow-up IQ <30 as compared to 57% of the control group.
- 9 of 19 children (47%) in the treatment group attended mainstream first-grade classes; no children in control group achieved this.

STUDY CONCLUSIONS

Children with ASD benefited significantly from intensive behavioral therapy with increased educational achievement and IQ. There was only rare improvement noted in those who did not receive this therapy.

COMMENTARY

This groundbreaking study first demonstrated a promising therapy for the treatment of autism, a disorder that previously had been considered untreatable and with poor prognosis. While each treatment group was small, the differences among groups were dramatic and provided hope for improvement in cognitive outcomes. While diagnostic criteria have since changed with the classification of ASD in the DSM-V, the old and new criteria largely overlap for children with significant impairment, similar to the study population. Many subsequent trials identified important treatment features for children with autism. These included early initiation of treatment services >25 hours per week, parent–teacher–physician involvement, and treatment of comorbid medical and psychiatric conditions.[1] They also highlighted potential benefits for early, intensive intervention to children with other risk factors, such as prematurity. The growth and success of this programming is a testament to the fact that, while treatment is time intensive and therefore expensive, it achieves lasting results in a child's development and may offer long-term public health cost saving.

Question

What is the most effective treatment for autism?

Answer

Early, intensive behavioral therapy has been shown to have the greatest impact on IQ and educational achievement.

Reference

1. Maglione MA, Gans D, Das L, et al. Nonmedical interventions for children with ASD: Recommended guidelines and further research needs. *Pediatrics.* 2012;130(Suppl 2):S169–S178.

PULMONOLOGY

84. Adenotonsillectomy for Obstructive Sleep Apnea
85. Hypertonic Saline in Cystic Fibrosis
86. Budesonide Treatment for Mild Asthma
87. Comparison of Oral Corticosteroid Doses in Asthma
88. Albuterol, Epinephrine, and Normal Saline for Bronchiolitis
89. Impact of Newborn Screening on Nutritional Status in Cystic Fibrosis
90. Route of Delivery of Beta-agonist Therapy
91. Risk of Asthma in Children With Early Wheezing

ADENOTONSILLECTOMY FOR OBSTRUCTIVE SLEEP APNEA

Eliza G. Stensland ■ Benjamin A. Nelson

Childhood Adenotonsillectomy Trial (CHAT). A Randomized Trial of Adenotonsillectomy for Childhood Sleep Apnea

Marcus CL, Moore RH, Rosen CL, et al. *N Engl J Med.* 2013;368(25):2366–2376

BACKGROUND
Obstructive sleep apnea (OSA) in children is associated with cognitive and behavioral disturbances. The most commonly identified risk factor for OSA is adenotonsillar hypertrophy, for which adenotonsillectomy is a common treatment. Prior studies demonstrated increased daytime sleepiness and learning problems in children with nighttime respiratory disturbances based upon parental surveys.[1] This was the first randomized controlled trial evaluating whether adenotonsillectomy was superior to watchful waiting in regard to cognition and behavior.

OBJECTIVES
To assess the effect of adenotonsillectomy on cognitive and behavioral function, quality of life, and sleep in pediatric patients with OSA.

METHODS
Single-blind, randomized controlled trial in 7 US sleep centers from 2008 to 2011.

Patients
464 children ages 5 to 9 years with mild-to-moderate OSA (apnea–hypopnea index [AHI] of ≥ 2 events per hour or an obstructive apnea index [OAI] of ≥ 1 event per hour). Select exclusion criteria: severe OSA with AHI >30, OAI of >20, recurrent tonsillitis, or use of medication for attention deficit hyperactivity disorder.

Intervention
Participants were randomized to adenotonsillectomy within 4 weeks or watchful waiting. They underwent polysomnographic (PSG) testing, cognitive and behavioral testing, and caregiver and teacher assessments at baseline and 7 months.

Outcomes
Primary outcome was change in the attention and executive function score using a previously established assessment tool. Secondary outcomes included change in OSA symptoms, daytime sleepiness, quality of life, PSG indices, and caregiver and teacher ratings of behavior.

KEY RESULTS

- Baseline scores in attention and executive function in both groups were similar to general population scores; surgical intervention did not significantly change these scores ($p = 0.16$).
- The adenotonsillectomy group had significantly improved caregiver ($p = 0.01$) and teacher ($p = 0.04$) behavioral ratings on the Conners Rating Scale.
- There was a significant increase in quality of life scores on a standardized tool in the children who underwent adenotonsillectomy ($p < 0.001$).
- More children in the adenotonsillectomy group showed improvement in PSG indices (79% vs. 46%, $p < 0.001$).

STUDY CONCLUSIONS

Although children with OSA who underwent adenotonsillectomy did not significantly improve attention or executive function as compared to controls, there was evidence to suggest improvement in some behavioral symptoms, quality of life, and PSG findings.

COMMENTARY

While this study demonstrated a significant improvement in behavior and PSG parameters among the treatment group, there were no differences in attention and executive function after 7 months, raising questions about the relative risks and benefits of surgical therapy. However, it is unclear whether the intervention group might have shown additional improvement in the long term. Although adenotonsillectomy is a viable treatment option for children with OSA, watchful waiting with close follow-up is also reasonable for patients with mild-to-moderate symptoms. These results cannot be extrapolated to children less than 5 years of age or those with severe OSA, which is significant since many patients are often first referred or noted to have tonsillar hypertrophy in early childhood.

Question

Does adenotonsillectomy benefit children with OSA?

Answer

In children ages 5 to 9 years with mild-to-moderate OSA, adenotonsillectomy does not improve scores of attention or executive function but does provide some improvement in behavior, quality of life, and abnormal PSG findings.

Reference

1. Goodwin JL, Kaemingk KL, Fregosi RF, et al. Clinical outcomes associated with sleep-disordered breathing in Caucasian and Hispanic children–the Tucson Children's Assessment of Sleep Apnea study (TuCASA). *Sleep.* 2003;26(5):587–591.

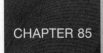

HYPERTONIC SALINE IN CYSTIC FIBROSIS

CHAPTER 85

Eliza G. Stensland ■ Benjamin A. Nelson

A Controlled Trial of Long-Term Inhaled Hypertonic Saline in Patients With Cystic Fibrosis
Elkins MR, Robinson M, Rose BR, et al. *N Engl J Med.* 2006;354(3):229–240

BACKGROUND
Approximately 30,000 US children are living with cystic fibrosis (CF).[1] In patients with CF, airway secretions are dry, leading to retained mucus, recurrent infection, and, ultimately, increased morbidity and mortality. Previous studies had shown that short-term administration of 7% hypertonic saline (HTS) improved mucociliary clearance and lung function. This study was the first to evaluate the impact of HTS on long-term outcomes in CF.

OBJECTIVES
To assess the long-term safety and efficacy of HTS treatments in patients with CF.

METHODS
Double-blind, parallel-group, randomized controlled trial in 16 hospitals in Australia from 2000 to 2003.

Patients
164 patients age >6 years (mean 18.7 ± 9.2) with clinically stable CF. Select exclusion criteria: pregnancy, breastfeeding, colonization with *Burkholderia cepacia*, cigarette smoking, prior HTS use, or nonroutine antibiotic use within 14 days.

Intervention
Participants received either HTS or 0.9% normal saline twice daily following broncho-dilator administration for 48 weeks. Patients received antibiotics as needed at physicians' discretion.

Outcomes
Primary outcome was linear rate of change of lung function measured as change in forced expiratory volume in 1 second (FEV_1), forced vital capacity (FVC), and forced expiratory flow at 25% to 75% of FVC at 0, 4, 12, 24, 36, and 48 weeks. Secondary outcomes included absolute lung function, pulmonary exacerbations (hemoptysis, dyspnea, and change in sputum), time free of exacerbations, antibiotic use, quality of life, and sputum pathogen analysis.

KEY RESULTS
- Although there was no statistical difference in the rate of lung function change between the 2 groups over the 48-week course ($p = 0.79$), absolute difference

in lung function was significant between the 2 groups when averaged over 4 to 48 weeks of treatment ($p = 0.03$).

- HTS group had significantly higher FVC (by 2.8%, 95% CI 0.4–5.2) and FEV_1 (by 3.2%, 95% CI 0.1–6.2) as compared to controls.
- HTS group had fewer pulmonary exacerbations (relative reduction 56%, $p = 0.02$), more participants without exacerbations requiring IV antibiotics (76% vs. 62%, $p = 0.03$), and fewer missed days of school/work (7 days vs. 24 days, $p <0.001$).
- HTS administration was not associated with changes in bacterial flora or inflammation as measured by sputum cytokines.

STUDY CONCLUSIONS

HTS preceded by bronchodilator therapy was a safe and effective adjunct treatment for patients with CF that improved lung function and reduced the incidence of pulmonary exacerbations.

COMMENTARY

At the time of this publication, there were no therapies targeting the mutated CFTR channel; therefore, this new therapy aimed at the underlying defect was groundbreaking. Limitations to applicability included lack of age-specific analyses and the Australian location due to differences in climate and bacterial pathogens. However, it illustrated benefits of longer treatment courses of HTS in CF, and led to widespread adoption of this relatively inexpensive therapy due to significantly fewer pulmonary exacerbations (a strong predictor of future morbidity and mortality) and decreased antibiotic use.[2]

Question

Do HTS treatments benefit patients with CF in the long term?

Answer

Yes, patients who are treated with HTS in addition to usual care over the course of 48 weeks have overall better lung function and fewer pulmonary exacerbations as compared to patients who receive isotonic saline treatments.

References

1. Cystic Fibrosis Foundation. Cystic fibrosis foundation patient registry 2012 annual data report. Bethesda, Maryland; 2013.
2. de Boer K, Vandemheen KL, Tullis E, et al. Exacerbation frequency and clinical outcomes in adult patients with cystic fibrosis. *Thorax.* 2011;66(8):680–685.

CHAPTER 86

BUDESONIDE TREATMENT FOR MILD ASTHMA

Eliza G. Stensland ■ Benjamin A. Nelson

Early Intervention With Budesonide in Mild Persistent Asthma: A Randomised, Double-Blind Trial

Pauwels RA, Pedersen S, Busse WW, et al. *Lancet.* 2003;361(9363):1071–1076

BACKGROUND
7 million US children have asthma; 1 in 5 of those have sought care for asthma in the emergency department and nearly half have missed school secondary to symptoms.[1] Multiple studies had demonstrated the utility of inhaled corticosteroids in treatment of chronic persistent asthma of all severities and that the majority of these benefits were gained if treatment was initiated within 2 years of symptom onset.[2] However, the benefit in the subset of patients with recent onset, persistent mild disease was unknown.

OBJECTIVES
To assess whether low-dose inhaled budesonide was beneficial in patients with <2 years of persistent mild asthma.

METHODS
Double-blind, randomized, placebo-controlled trial conducted across 499 sites in 32 countries from 1996 to 1998.

Patients
7,241 patients ages 5 to 66 years (3,195 age ≤17 years) with persistent mild asthma (reversible airway obstruction on spirometry and symptoms of wheeze, cough, dyspnea or chest tightening ≥1 time per week but not daily for <2 years). Select exclusion criteria: >30 days of corticosteroid treatment or >1 depot corticosteroid injection annually.

Intervention
Budesonide (400 mcg if ≥11 years old, 200 mcg if <11 years old at the start of the study) or placebo in addition to usual asthma therapy. Follow-up visits with spirometry occurred periodically for 3 years.

Outcomes
Primary outcome was time to first severe asthma-related event (hospital admission, emergency treatment for worsening symptoms, or death). Secondary outcomes included number of asthma-free days and time to introduction of supplemental inhaled or oral steroid treatment.

KEY RESULTS

- Budesonide reduced the risk of first severe asthma-related event (hazard ratio 0.56, 95% CI 0.45–0.71); fewer patients on budesonide had life-threatening asthma events ($p = 0.009$).
- Budesonide group had more symptom-free days ($p < 0.0001$) and received fewer oral corticosteroid courses (OR 0.59, 95% CI 0.53–0.67).
- Children ages 5-10 on budesonide had improved post-bronchodilator forced expiratory volume in 1 second after 3 years ($p = 0.004$); this was not seen in adolescents.
- Children ages 5-15 receiving budesonide had decreased growth rates compared to placebo (mean difference –0.43 cm/y, 95% CI –0.54 to –0.32).

STUDY CONCLUSIONS

Early initiation of inhaled budesonide for patients with persistent mild asthma delayed onset of first severe exacerbation and improved overall control.

COMMENTARY

This study laid the groundwork for early introduction of inhaled corticosteroids in patients with less severe disease, thereby greatly improving outcomes and quality of life. While a significant improvement in lung function was not seen in adolescents, this could be due to the natural history of the disease, thus showing a diminished overall difference. The inclusion of adults limits the study power when applied to children, suggesting a need for future pediatric studies. Nonetheless, the National Asthma Education and Prevention Program now recommends inhaled corticosteroids as first-line therapy in all patients with persistent asthma.[3]

Question

Does early treatment with budesonide in patients with mild asthma improve disease control?

Answer

Yes, once daily treatment with budesonide in patients with persistent mild asthma reduces the risk of severe exacerbations and need for corticosteroids.

References

1. Centers for Disease Control and Prevention, National Asthma Control Program. Asthma's impact on the nation. Available at: http://www.cdc.gov/asthma/impacts_nation/asthmafactsheet.pdf. Accessed on July 15, 2015.
2. Selroos O, Pietinalho A, Lofroos AB, et al. Effect of early vs. late intervention with inhaled corticosteroid in asthma. *Chest*. 1995;108(5):1228–1234.
3. National Asthma Education and Prevention Program. Expert Panel Report 3 (EPR-3): Guidelines for the diagnosis and management of asthma—summary report 2007. *J Allergy Clin Immunol*. 2007;120 (5 Suppl):S94–S138.

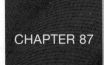

COMPARISON OF ORAL CORTICOSTEROID DOSES IN ASTHMA

CHAPTER 87

Max Rubinstein ■ Benjamin A. Nelson

Adverse Behavioral Effects of Treatment for Acute Exacerbation of Asthma in Children: A Comparison of Two Doses of Oral Steroids

Kayani S, Shannon DC. *Chest.* 2002;122(2):624–628

BACKGROUND

In the US in 2010–11, there were 15.5 million outpatient visits for asthma exacerbations and 1.5 million ED visits.[1] Many of these patients are prescribed oral corticosteroids, with children receiving proportionally higher weight-based doses than adults, between 1-2 mg/kg/d. There was concern that higher doses could precipitate behavioral or psychiatric issues, but it was unknown whether these doses were necessary to adequately treat asthma exacerbations in children. This study sought to investigate the effects of varying oral corticosteroid doses.

OBJECTIVES

To determine the relative benefits and adverse effects of different doses of oral corticosteroids in children with mild asthma exacerbations.

METHODS

Double-blind, randomized trial at a single US center.

Patients

86 outpatients ages 2 to 16 years with mild persistent asthma on inhaled corticosteroids evaluated for exacerbations (defined as cough, shortness of breath, or persistent wheeze after 3 consecutive albuterol treatments in 1 hour). Select exclusion criteria: oral corticosteroid therapy within 2 weeks of presentation, underlying attention deficit hyperactivity disorder, or psychiatric illness.

Intervention

Comparison of a 5-day course of 1 mg/kg/d vs. 2 mg/kg/d of prednisone or prednisolone, in addition to doubling inhaled corticosteroid dose and using albuterol every 6 hours. A parental questionnaire was administered by telephone 5 days and 2 weeks after treatment.

Outcomes

Primary outcome was adverse effects of corticosteroid treatment. Secondary outcome was efficacy of corticosteroid therapy.

KEY RESULTS

- Anxiety was significantly increased in patients receiving 2 mg/kg/d of corticosteroids (RR 4.5, 95% CI 1.0–19.6; number needed to harm [NNH] 6.1, 95% CI 38.4–3.3).

- Aggressive behavior was increased in patients on higher dose of corticosteroids (0 vs. 9 patients, NNH 4.8, 95% CI 11.2–3).
- All patients in the study except 1 child in the 2 mg/kg/d cohort had complete asthma symptom resolution at 2 weeks.
- No patients required hospital admission.

STUDY CONCLUSIONS

Compared to 1 mg/kg/d dosing of oral corticosteroids, 2 mg/kg/d dosing increased the risk of adverse behavioral side effects in children with mild asthma exacerbations without producing an incremental benefit in symptom resolution.

COMMENTARY

Before this study, there was little evidence to recommend specific doses of oral corticosteroids for treatment of mild asthma exacerbations in children. This study demonstrated that higher doses increased the risk of psychiatric adverse effects without increasing efficacy. Recent literature also suggests that 3-day courses of corticosteroids are equivalent to 5-day courses in the management of outpatient exacerbations.[2] It is important to note that this paper excluded children requiring hospitalization, raising the possibility that higher corticosteroid dosing may be useful in this sicker population. Because of this limitation, the 2007 National Institutes of Health guidelines for the management of pediatric asthma exacerbations state that providers may give 1-2 mg/kg/d, despite the lack of evidence for increased efficacy of higher doses of corticosteroids for severe asthma exacerbations.[3]

Question

What dose of oral corticosteroids is appropriate for treating outpatient asthma exacerbations?

Answer

Evidence suggests use of 1 mg/kg/d of oral corticosteroids is as efficacious as 2 mg/kg/d, with decreased behavioral adverse effects.

References

1. Centers for Disease Control and Prevention. "Asthma," FastStats. Available at: http://www.cdc.gov/nchs/fastats/asthma.htm. Modified on January 20, 2015. Accessed on May 1, 2015.
2. Chang AB, Clark R, Sloots TP, et al. A 5- versus 3-day course of oral corticosteroids for children with asthma exacerbations who are not hospitalised: A randomised controlled trial. *Med J Aust.* 2008;189(6):306–310.
3. National Asthma Education and Prevention Program. Expert Panel Report 3 (EPR-3): Guidelines for the diagnosis and management of asthma—summary report 2007. *J Allergy Clin Immunol.* 2007;120 (5 Suppl):S94–S138.

CHAPTER 88

ALBUTEROL, EPINEPHRINE, AND NORMAL SALINE FOR BRONCHIOLITIS

Max Rubinstein ■ Benjamin A. Nelson

A Randomized, Controlled Trial of the Effectiveness of Nebulized Therapy With Epinephrine Compared With Albuterol and Saline in Infants Hospitalized for Acute Viral Bronchiolitis

Patel H, Platt RW, Pekeles GS, et al. *J Pediatr.* 2002;141(6):818–824

BACKGROUND

Approximately 100,000 infants in the US are admitted annually for bronchiolitis, with a total cost of $1.7 billion.[1] Despite its high incidence, there is a frustrating lack of effective disease-specific therapy. Nebulized albuterol and epinephrine are often trialed to treat infants' work of breathing and hypoxemia. This study sought to assess their effectiveness in reducing length of stay, thereby reducing bronchiolitis' impact on healthcare costs.

OBJECTIVES

To compare length of stay in infants admitted with bronchiolitis treated with nebulized albuterol, epinephrine, and normal saline (placebo).

METHODS

Double-blind, randomized, placebo-controlled, parallel-group trial in a single hospital in Canada from 1998 to 2000.

Patients

149 infants age <12 months hospitalized with clinically defined bronchiolitis (oxygen saturation <95% on room air, poor feeding, lethargy, sustained tachypnea, or other concerning signs). Select exclusion criteria: history of wheezing, bronchopulmonary dysplasia, and intensive care unit admission.

Intervention

Randomization to nebulized racemic epinephrine (EPI), albuterol (ALB) or normal saline (PLAC) every 1 to 6 hours at physicians' discretion. All infants were scored with the Respiratory Distress Assessment Instrument (RDAI).

Outcomes

Primary outcome was length of hospital stay (LOS). Secondary outcomes included time from admission until normal oxygenation, adequate fluid intake, and minimal respiratory distress.

KEY RESULTS

- Of 149 infants (mean age 4.3 ± 3.1 months), 71% had respiratory syncytial virus (RSV).

- There was no significant difference in length of stay among the 3 groups (EPI 59.8 hours, ALB 61.4 hours, and PLAC 63.3 hours, $p = 0.95$).
- Albuterol and epinephrine were equally associated with mild adverse effects (transient tachycardia, mild hypertension, and slight tremor).
- There was no difference among groups in mean time to achieving normal oxygenation, adequate fluid intake, minimal respiratory distress, or ability to space nebulizer administration to less than every 4 hours.
- 8 patients returned to the emergency department after discharge (1 in EPI group, 3 in ALB group, and 4 in PLAC group); 3 patients were readmitted, all from the placebo group.

STUDY CONCLUSIONS

The use of nebulized epinephrine or albuterol as compared to normal saline did not significantly shorten the hospital length of stay in infants with viral bronchiolitis. There was also no improvement in secondary measures of clinical status.

COMMENTARY

This study adds to the body of literature demonstrating a lack of efficacy from routine use of nebulized medications and informed the 2014 American Academy of Pediatrics (AAP) guidelines recommending against their administration.[1] Of note, these recommendations include hypertonic saline in those pharmacologic agents that lack evidence for use. Despite these guidelines, recent data show bronchodilators are given to over half of patients with bronchiolitis.[2] It is important to note that this study's data excluded older patients and those with prior wheezing episodes, allowing the possibility that certain subpopulations of infants with bronchiolitis may have an Immunoglobulin E–mediated process that could respond more vigorously to nebulized medications. However, a clearly responsive subpopulation has yet to be definitively identified.

Question

Should albuterol or nebulized epinephrine be routinely used in infants with viral bronchiolitis?

Answer

No. Current evidence does not support the use of these medications in this population.

References

1. Ralston SL, Lieberthal AS, Meissner HC, et al. Clinical practice guideline: The diagnosis, management, and prevention of bronchiolitis. *Pediatrics.* 2014;134(5):e1474–e1502.
2. Parikh K, Hall M, Teach SJ, et al. Bronchiolitis management before and after the AAP guidelines. *Pediatrics.* 2014;133(1):e1–e7.

CHAPTER 89

IMPACT OF NEWBORN SCREENING ON NUTRITIONAL STATUS IN CYSTIC FIBROSIS

Max Rubinstein ■ Benjamin A. Nelson

Early Diagnosis of Cystic Fibrosis Through Neonatal Screening Prevents Severe Malnutrition and Improves Long-Term Growth

Farrell PM, Kosorok MR, Rock MJ, et al. *Pediatrics.* 2001;107(1):1–13

BACKGROUND

Cystic fibrosis (CF) was historically difficult to diagnose; in 1996, the mean age of diagnosis in the US was 4.8 years. Delays in starting appropriate treatment are associated with more severe lung disease, malnutrition, and earlier mortality. Neonatal CF screening (via immunoreactive trypsinogen [IRT] measurement techniques) was first introduced in the 1970s and optimized with genetic testing in the 1990s, leading to early identification of most children with CF. However, at the time of this study, widespread early screening had not been adopted due to lack of evidence of potential health benefits.

OBJECTIVES

To determine the incidence of CF and assess the benefits and risks of early CF diagnosis through newborn screening.

METHODS

Randomized clinical trial at multiple centers in 1 US state from 1985 to 1994.

Patients

650,341 newborns were enrolled. Select exclusion criterion: meconium ileus.

Intervention

IRT levels were obtained on all specimens, with the addition of ΔF508 mutation DNA testing in 1991. In the early screening group, positivity of either test was confirmed with sweat testing. In the control group, results were stored blinded until parental request for results or until patient reached age 4. After diagnosis, patients were encouraged to eat high-calorie/high-fat diets, provided vitamins and supplements, and followed closely for up to 13 years. Assessments for pancreatic insufficiency, fat malabsorption, and vitamin deficiency were performed.

Outcomes

Primary outcomes were age at diagnosis of CF and subsequent dietary intake, and growth measures of both screened and control patients.

KEY RESULTS
- CF incidence (confirmed by sweat test) was 1:4,189 (95% CI 3,603–4,930).
- Screened patients were diagnosed earlier than control patients (13 ± 37 weeks vs. 100 ± 117 weeks, p <0.001).
- Screened patients had greater percentiles for head circumference (52% vs. 35%, p = 0.003), height (44% vs. 26%, p <0.001), and weight at diagnosis (35% vs. 24%, p <0.001).
- Despite similar nutritional therapy to screened patients, control patients were more likely to be <10th percentile for both height (p = 0.007) and weight (p = 0.004) for several years after diagnosis.

STUDY CONCLUSIONS
Early diagnosis and treatment of CF were associated with significant nutritional advantages that persisted for years beyond diagnosis.

COMMENTARY
Given the relationship between poor anthropometric indices and morbidity in patients with CF, this study argued strongly for inclusion of CF in newborn screening panels prior to symptom onset. Of note, a significant difference was noted between the 2 groups with respect to genotype and likely phenotype of CF, and there were more severely affected children in the early diagnosis group. European studies have suggested that early diagnosis is associated with improved lung function, although US studies are more ambiguous.[1,2] Economic analyses have also associated early diagnosis with decreased cumulative cost of care.[3] As a result of these data, CF testing is now part of newborn screening in all US states.

Question
Does early diagnosis of CF have clinical benefits?

Answer
Yes, early diagnosis and treatment is associated with improved growth and nutritional outcomes in childhood.

References
1. Farrell PM, Li Z, Kosorok MR, et al. Bronchopulmonary disease in children with cystic fibrosis after early or delayed diagnosis. *Am J Respir Crit Care Med.* 2003;168(9):1100–1108.
2. Dankert-Roelse JE, Mérelle ME. Review of outcomes of neonatal screening for cystic fibrosis versus non-screening in Europe. *J Pediatr.* 2005;147(3 Suppl):S15–S20.
3. Sims EJ, Mugford M, Clark A, et al. Economic implications of newborn screening for cystic fibrosis: A cost of illness retrospective cohort study. *Lancet.* 2007;369(9568):1187–1195.

CHAPTER 90

ROUTE OF DELIVERY OF BETA-AGONIST THERAPY

Max Rubinstein ■ Benjamin A. Nelson

Randomized Trial of Salbutamol via Metered-Dose Inhaler With Spacer Versus Nebulizer for Acute Wheezing in Children Less Than 2 Years of Age

Rubilar L, Castro-Rodriguez JA, Girardi G. *Pediatr Pulmonol.* 2000;29(4):264–269

BACKGROUND

Metered-dose inhalers (MDI) with spacers deliver more medication directly to the lungs, and offer ease of use, portability, and cost effectiveness. However, in young children requiring treatment for wheezing, nebulized route of administration was utilized near universally.[1] Studies in older patients suggested equivalency of beta-2 (β2) agonist administered via MDI vs. nebulizers (NEB); data were limited in young children.

OBJECTIVES

To compare the efficacy of β2-agonist (salbutamol) administration via NEB vs. MDI with spacer in children <2 years of age.

METHODS

Single-blind, randomized clinical trial in a pediatric emergency department (ED) in Chile during a single winter.

Patients

123 children ages 1 to 24 months presenting with moderate-to-severe wheezing characterized by a standardized score. Select exclusion criteria: pneumonia; chronic pulmonary, cardiac, or neurologic disease; foreign body aspiration.

Intervention

Administration of salbutamol for 1 hour either as 0.25 mg/kg (maximum 5 mg) of 0.5% solution via NEB every 20 minutes or 2 puffs of 100 mcg/puff via MDI with spacer every 10 minutes (maximum 5 doses). Patients with subsequent scores >5 received another hour of the same treatment, supplemental oxygen, and betamethasone 0.5 mg/kg IM. Patients with persistent scores >5 were admitted.

Outcomes

Primary outcome was severity of respiratory distress by clinical score (including respiratory rate, wheezing severity, cyanosis, accessory muscle use). Secondary outcomes included adverse events and hospital admissions.

KEY RESULTS

- After 1 hour of treatment, 90% of MDI group scored ≤5 compared to 71% of NEB group (OR 3.9, 95% CI 1.5–10.4). There was no persistent significant difference at 2 hours.
- In children age <6 months, 96% of MDI group and 73% of NEB group scored ≤5 after 1 hour ($p = 0.035$).
- Changes in clinical score from admission to 1 hour after treatment showed a difference between children in the NEB group vs. MDI group (mean ± SD, 2.9 ± 1.2 vs. 3.8 ± 1.0, respectively, p <0.0001); changes from admission to the second hour after treatment were 4.0 ± 0.8 in the NEB group vs. 5.3 ± 0.8 in the MDI group (p <0.002).
- Children with history of multiple wheezing episodes also had faster responses in clinical score with MDI use ($p = 0.03$).

STUDY CONCLUSIONS

Children <2 years old with moderate-to-severe wheezing responded faster to β2-agonist delivery via MDI compared to NEB though the advantage was not sustained.

COMMENTARY

This study was one of the earliest to support efficacy of MDIs even in young children. Notably, this study was single blinded, and excluded children with severe wheezing. However, subsequent double-blind placebo-controlled trials found similar results, and cost-analysis studies demonstrated savings with ED use of MDIs for mild-to-moderate exacerbations.[2,3] Despite this evidence, the continued variation in practice may be due to parental and clinician concern regarding successful coordination of MDI administration.

Question

Can MDIs be used effectively in wheezing children <2 years old?

Answer

Yes, β2-agonists given via MDI with spacer are as effective as those delivered via nebulization and may result in faster symptom resolution.

References

1. Bloomberg GR. Recurrent wheezing illness in preschool-aged children: Assessment and management in primary care practice. *Postgrad Med.* 2009;121(5):48–55.
2. Delgado A, Chou KJ, Silver EJ, et al. Nebulizers vs metered-dose inhalers with spacers for bronchodilator therapy to treat wheezing in children aged 2 to 24 months in a pediatric emergency department. *Arch Pediatr Adolesc Med.* 2003;157(1):76–80.
3. Doan Q, Shefrin A, Johnson D. Cost-effectiveness of metered-dose inhalers for asthma exacerbations in the pediatric emergency department. *Pediatrics.* 2011;127(5):e1105–e1111.

RISK OF ASTHMA IN CHILDREN WITH EARLY WHEEZING

CHAPTER 91

Max Rubinstein ■ Benjamin A. Nelson

Asthma and Wheezing in the First Six Years of Life. The Group Health Medical Associates

Martinez FD, Wright AL, Taussig LM, et al. *N Engl J Med.* 1995;332(3):133–138

BACKGROUND

In the US, up to 1/3 of children will have at least 1 wheezing episode by age 3.[1] To improve discussions surrounding prognosis and treatment with families, a better understanding of both the pathogenesis and correlation of early wheezing to asthma development was needed. This study was one of the first to follow children longitudinally from infancy onward.

OBJECTIVES

To document the natural history of early childhood wheezing and identify predictors for future development of asthma.

METHODS

Prospective cohort study in a single US center from 1980 to 1990.

Patients

826 children enrolled at birth in the Tucson Children's Respiratory Study and who completed follow-up at 3 and 6 years. Select exclusion criteria: none.

Intervention

Baseline family characteristics were collected at enrollment, with follow-up questionnaires regarding symptoms of wheeze and allergic rhinitis. Children were evaluated for all respiratory illness(es). Immunoglobulin E (IgE) levels, pulmonary function tests, and skin testing were obtained within the first year and at 6 years.

Outcomes

Primary outcome was wheezing history divided into 4 categories: no wheezing, early transient wheezing (resolved by age 3), late-onset wheezing (starting after age 3), and persistent wheezing (starting before age 3 and still noted at age 6). Secondary outcomes were risk factors associated with wheezing in each subgroup.

KEY RESULTS

- By age 6, 51.5% of children had never wheezed, 19.9% had early transient wheezing, 15% had late-onset wheezing, and 13.7% had persistent wheezing.
- 59% of children who wheezed in their first 3 years no longer had episodes by age 6.

- Children with persistent wheezing had higher IgE levels at 9 months ($p = 0.02$) and at 6 years ($p < 0.01$) than children who had never wheezed.
- Children were more likely to develop persistent wheezing if they had eczema (OR 2.4, 95% CI 1.3–4.6), allergic rhinitis (OR 2.0, 95% CI 1.2–3.2), maternal asthma (OR 4.1, 95% CI 2.1–7.9), Hispanic ethnicity (OR 3.0, 95% CI 1.6–5.5), or positive maternal smoking status (OR 2.3, 95% CI 1.2–4.4).

STUDY CONCLUSIONS

Most young children with wheezing were not at increased risk of subsequently developing asthma. Allergic rhinitis, eczema, exposure to tobacco smoke, elevated IgE, Hispanic ethnicity, and maternal asthma history were independent risk factors for persistent wheezing.

COMMENTARY

This study allowed pediatricians to better distinguish between young children with self-limited wheezing and those who would develop more long-standing symptoms. It remains unclear if certain infections or other modifiable risk factors are associated with the development of asthma. Subsequent studies have suggested that certain viruses are associated with an increased asthma incidence; however, wheezing with these infections may simply be markers of a child at increased risk of developing asthma rather than a causal mechanism.[2] No treatment has been shown to prevent high-risk patients from developing asthma.[3]

Question

Which wheezing infants are likely to develop asthma later in life?

Answer

Children with eczema, allergic rhinitis, maternal asthma history, maternal smoking history, elevated IgE, or Hispanic ethnicity are at increased risk.

References

1. Eldeirawi K, Persky VW. History of ear infections and prevalence of asthma in a national sample of children aged 2 to 11 years: The Third National Health and Nutrition Examination Survey, 1988 to 1994. *Chest.* 2004;125(5):1685–1692.
2. Carroll KN, Wu P, Gebretsadik T, et al. Season of infant bronchiolitis and estimates of subsequent risk and burden of early childhood asthma. *J Allergy Clin Immunol.* 2009;123(4):964–966.
3. Bisgaard H, Bønnelykke K. Long-term studies of the natural history of asthma in childhood. *J Allergy Clin Immunol.* 2010;126(2):187–197.

RENAL

92. Antimicrobial Prophylaxis for Children With
Vesicoureteral Reflux
93. Mortality Associated With Acute Kidney Injury
94. Impact of Blood Pressure Control on Progression
of Renal Failure
95. Outcomes After Acute Kidney Injury
96. Response to Prednisone in Nephrotic Syndrome

ANTIMICROBIAL PROPHYLAXIS FOR CHILDREN WITH VESICOURETERAL REFLUX

Michael Epstein ■ Avram Z. Traum

Antimicrobial Prophylaxis for Children With Vesicoureteral Reflux

RIVUR (Randomized Intervention for Children With Vesicoureteral Reflux) Trial Investigators, Hoberman A, Greenfield SP, et al. *N Engl J Med.* 2014;370(25):2367–2376

BACKGROUND

Vesicoureteral reflux (VUR) is present in 1/3 of children with febrile urinary tract infections (UTI) and is a known risk factor for recurrent infections. UTIs and reflux can lead to renal scarring and chronic kidney disease, also known as reflux nephropathy. Despite this, data on efficacy of antibiotic prophylaxis in VUR were inconsistent and scarce. RIVUR was the first large trial with rigorous methodology to attempt establishment of an evidence-based standard of care.

OBJECTIVES

To determine the efficacy of long-term antibiotic prophylaxis in preventing UTI recurrence and renal scarring in children with VUR.

METHODS

Double-blind, randomized, placebo-controlled trial in 19 US centers from 2007 to 2011.

Patients

607 children ages 2 to 71 months with grade I–IV VUR diagnosed after a first or second UTI. Select exclusion criteria: other urologic anomalies.

Intervention

Daily prophylaxis with trimethoprim-sulfamethoxazole (TMP-SMX; 3 mg/kg TMP component) or placebo for 24 months. Participants underwent urine cultures when having fever or dysuria, baseline and annual nuclear medicine scans to assess for renal scarring, and rectal swabs at the beginning and end of the study to document antibiotic susceptibilities of *Escherichia coli* isolates.

Outcomes

Primary outcome was febrile or symptomatic UTI recurrence (pyuria, positive urine culture, or urinary tract symptoms). Secondary outcomes were renal scarring and antimicrobial resistance, as well as prophylaxis failure (composite of UTI recurrence and renal scarring).

KEY RESULTS

- Children receiving prophylaxis were less likely to develop UTI than those receiving placebo (hazard ratio [HR] 0.50, $p < 0.001$).

- In number needed to treat (NNT) analysis, 8 children (95% CI 5–16) would need 2 years of prophylaxis to prevent 1 UTI.
- In subgroup analysis, prophylaxis reduced UTI risk in children with febrile index infections (HR 0.41, 95% CI 0.26–0.64) and baseline bowel/bladder dysfunction (HR 0.21, CI 0.08–0.58).
- At the end of the study, there were no significant differences between the 2 groups in new renal scars from baseline ($p = 0.94$) or overall renal scarring ($p = 0.55$).
- Resistance to TMP-SMX was significantly more common in UTI recurrences among those on prophylaxis as compared to those on placebo (63% vs. 19%, $p < 0.001$).

STUDY CONCLUSIONS

Children with VUR diagnosed after initial UTI were less likely to develop UTI recurrence if given TMP-SMX prophylaxis, but did not exhibit a significant difference in renal scarring.

COMMENTARY

Despite initial hopes, the RIVUR trial did not establish an unambiguous standard of care. The study was not powered to show a difference in rates of scarring between groups, and was further hampered by the relatively short follow-up period (2 years) and low proportion (8.3%) of cohort subjects with grade IV reflux. TMP-SMX prophylaxis was demonstrated to be efficacious in preventing UTI recurrence, although the clinical significance is questionable given the high infection-free rates in both groups and the high NNT to prevent 1 infection over a 2-year period. Furthermore, there was a higher rate of TMP-SMX resistance in the prophylaxis arm, which represents a potentially serious drawback as these patients will continue to be at high risk of UTI requiring future antibiotic therapy. Therefore, the RIVUR trial did not clearly demonstrate that the benefits of antibiotic prophylaxis in children with low-to-moderate grade (I–III) VUR clearly outweigh the risks.

Question

Should children with UTIs who are found to have VUR receive long-term antimicrobial prophylaxis to prevent recurrence?

Answer

Unfortunately, a definitive answer remains elusive. Antimicrobial prophylaxis is efficacious at preventing recurrent infections, but it increases antibiotic resistance in patients' flora and may not lead to improved clinical outcomes.

CHAPTER 93	# MORTALITY ASSOCIATED WITH ACUTE KIDNEY INJURY

Michael Epstein ■ Avram Z. Traum

Serum Creatinine as Stratified in the RIFLE Score for Acute Kidney Injury is Associated With Mortality and Length of Stay for Children in the Pediatric Intensive Care Unit

Schneider J, Khemani R, Grushkin C, et al. *Crit Care Med.* 2010;38(3):933–939

BACKGROUND

Acute kidney injury (AKI) is associated with poor outcomes in adult and pediatric intensive care units (PICU). However, prevalence of AKI in critically ill patients was not well characterized, in part due to lack of an accepted definition. To address this, the Acute Dialysis Quality Initiative introduced the adult RIFLE criteria in 2002. Severity is stratified by relative increase in serum creatinine compared to baseline: "Risk" (1.5×), "Injury" (2×), and "Failure" (3×). Outcomes are stratified into "Loss" and "End stage renal disease" (ESRD). Multiple studies subsequently validated this RIFLE score and it quickly gained acceptance; this study sought to validate the criteria in children.

OBJECTIVES

To assess the ability of the RIFLE criteria to characterize AKI and predict outcomes in critically ill children.

METHODS

Retrospective analysis of prospectively collected cohort data in 1 US PICU from 2003 to 2007.

Patients

3,396 separate PICU admissions. Select exclusion criteria: age <30 days or >21 years, pre-existing renal insufficiency, ESRD.

Intervention

RIFLE stratifications of R, I, or F were assigned based upon serum creatinine at baseline (patient's creatinine ≤6 months ago or normal for age/gender), within 24 hours of admission, and throughout ICU stay. Stratifications of L and E were used as end points.

Outcomes

Primary outcome was mortality. Secondary outcome was PICU length of stay.

KEY RESULTS

• AKI prevalence during hospitalization was 10% (339/3,396); 5.7% (194/3,396) had AKI on admission.

- Nearly half of all patients had peak serum creatinine within 24 hours of ICU admission, while about 75% achieved their maximum RIFLE score by ICU day 7.
- Mortality was 32% (OR 9.17, CI 6.51–12.91) for those presenting with AKI and 30% (OR 11.43, CI 8.47–15.38) for those who later developed AKI, as compared to only 3.7% in those without AKI.
- Progression from no AKI on admission to R, I, and F increased the mortality OR to 5.8 (CI 3.08–10.87), 14.24 (CI 7.52–27), and 21 (CI 9.9–44.64), respectively. If AKI was present on admission, R/I/F stratification did not change mortality rate.
- Length of stay was increased for those with AKI as compared to patients with normal renal function on admission (5 vs. 1.9 days, p<0.01) as well as those who developed AKI during PICU stay as compared to those with normal renal function (p vs 1.8, p<0.01).

STUDY CONCLUSIONS

In children, AKI on admission or during PICU stay was associated with increased mortality and length of stay. The RIFLE score was predictive of degree of increased mortality for those patients that developed AKI during their stay, but not for those presenting with AKI.

COMMENTARY
This study validated the use of RIFLE criteria for hospital-acquired AKI in critically ill children. It was notable for its large size, more representative cohort than previous trials, and stringent terminology. It encourages PICU providers to identify and treat even small increases in serum creatinine as early as possible to reduce mortality. It also supported more widespread use of pRIFLE, the pediatric modification of the criteria that utilizes creatinine clearance, as a standardized approach for grading AKI both clinically and for research purposes.

Question

Are there criteria for classifying clinically relevant outcomes for patients with AKI in the PICU?

Answer

Yes. The RIFLE criteria stratify AKI based on proportional rise in serum creatinine; higher scores are associated with worse outcomes and longer PICU stays.

CHAPTER 94

IMPACT OF BLOOD PRESSURE CONTROL ON PROGRESSION OF RENAL FAILURE

Michael Epstein ■ Avram Z. Traum

Strict Blood-Pressure Control and Progression of Renal Failure in Children

ESCAPE (Effect of Strict Blood Pressure Control and ACE Inhibition on the Progression of CRF in Pediatric Patients) Trial Group, Wühl E, Trivelli A, et al. *N Engl J Med.* 2009; 361(17):1639–1650

BACKGROUND

In adults, tight blood pressure (BP) control, particularly through use of angiotensin converting enzyme inhibitors (ACEi), can delay the progression of chronic kidney disease (CKD) to end stage renal disease (ESRD). Prior to this study, similar efficacy had not been demonstrated in pediatrics, despite the high prevalence of hypertension in children with CKD and its known contribution to ESRD development. Furthermore, benchmarks for optimal BP control had not been established.

OBJECTIVES

To compare conventional vs. intensive BP control on the rate of progression of CKD to ESRD in children.

METHODS

Randomized controlled trial at 33 European sites from 1998 to 2001.

Patients

385 children ages 3 to 18 with stage II–IV CKD (glomerular filtration rate [GFR] of 15 to 80 mL/min/1.73 m^2 body surface area) with hypertension (24-hour mean arterial pressure [MAP] >95th percentile and/or an antihypertensive prescription). Select exclusion criteria: renal artery stenosis, kidney transplant, or other severe organ dysfunction.

Intervention

Target-intensive BP goal of <50th percentile compared to conventional goal of 50th to 95th percentile. Both groups received an ACEi (ramipril, 6 mg/m^2) and additional non-renin–angiotensin–aldosterone system (RAAS) antihypertensives as needed.

KEY RESULTS

- Fewer patients in the intensive group had reached the primary end points by 5 years than in the conventional group: 25.2% (46/182) vs. 36.3% (69/190), p = 0.02. Risk of progression was reduced in the intensive group (hazard ratio 0.65, 95% CI 0.44–0.94).

- Mean systolic and diastolic BPs were both reduced equally in each group ($p = 0.22$, $p = 0.5$, respectively).
- 50% reduction in proteinuria within the first 2 months of ACEi therapy correlated with a delay in CKD progression in both groups ($p = 0.005$); proteinuria gradually increased back to baseline by 36 months.
- There was no significant difference in type or frequency of adverse events, or in study withdrawal, between the 2 groups.

Outcomes

Primary outcome was time to 50% reduction in GFR or ESRD. Secondary end points included changes in BP, GFR, and proteinuria.

STUDY CONCLUSIONS

Targeting BP control to a more intensive goal of <50th percentile delayed CKD progression in children more efficaciously than a more conservative BP goal.

COMMENTARY

This study showed that intensified BP targets for children conferred a further delay in CKD progression despite the fact that the intensified group had only a modestly lower than the conventional group (a phenomenon that the authors attribute to the high background efficacy of ramipril). This finding implies that either the small differences in BP control between groups, and/or additional effects of antihypertensives beyond BP lowering, was of lasting benefit to children with CKD. Importantly, this study demonstrated, for the first time, the safety and efficacy of targeting BPs in a lower range of normal for children with CKD. In 2009, the European Society of Hypertension recommended a target BP below the 75th percentile for children with CKD (without proteinuria) and below 50% in those with proteinuria.[1]

Question

How does BP management affect disease progression in children with CKD?

Answer

Intensively targeting lower BP (<50th percentile) with ACEi combined with other antihypertensive agents confers a greater benefit in terms of disease progression than a more conventional target of 50th to 95th percentile.

Reference

1. Lurbe E, Cifkova R, Cruickshank JK, et al. Management of high blood pressure in children and adolescents: Recommendations of the European Society of Hypertension. *J Hypertens.* 2009;27(9):1719–1742.

CHAPTER 95

OUTCOMES AFTER ACUTE KIDNEY INJURY

Michael Epstein ■ Avram Z. Traum

3–5 Year Longitudinal Follow-Up of Pediatric Patients After Acute Renal Failure
Askenazi DJ, Feig DI, Graham NM, et al. *Kidney Int.* 2006;69(1):184–189

BACKGROUND

Acute renal failure (ARF), now known as acute kidney injury (AKI), is a significant cause of morbidity and mortality among hospitalized children. A 2005 study from these researchers demonstrated 29% mortality during the initial hospitalization for children with AKI, with higher mortality rates in ICU patients and those receiving renal replacement therapy (RRT).[1] Among survivors, 68% had completely recovered renal function by discharge and only 5% had end stage renal disease (ESRD). However, long-term outcomes in the children with AKI who survived hospitalization were not known until this follow-up study.

OBJECTIVES

To measure 3- to 5-year patient and renal survival after AKI.

METHODS

Retrospective cross-sectional/cohort (blended methodology) study at a single US center from 1998 to 2001.

Patients

174 children surviving to hospital discharge with diagnosis of ARF listed on discharge summary. Select exclusion criteria: chronic kidney disease or previous transplant.

Intervention

Parents, physicians, and medical records were queried to determine survival. A subset of patients was then evaluated for signs of renal injury (microalbuminuria, decreased glomerular filtration rate [GFR], hematuria, and hypertension) over a 3- to 5-year follow-up period.

Outcomes

Primary outcomes were mortality and renal survival (i.e., nonprogression to ESRD). Secondary outcomes included GFR, microalbuminuria, hypertension, and quality of life.

KEY RESULTS

- 3- to 5-year survival was 79.9% (139/174). 68.5% (24/35) of deaths occurred ≤12 months after hospitalization.

- No significant differences in mortality were observed for patients with ICU vs. no ICU stay, RRT vs. no RRT, or renal/urologic comorbidities, all of which had been significant predictors of mortality during initial hospitalization.
- There was 90.8% (158/174) renal survival at 3 to 5 years. This was less likely in those with primary renal/urologic conditions (68.6% [24/35]), but need for ICU or RRT was not predictive.
- Of the 29 patients evaluated further in the cohort, 6 (20.9%) had hypertension and 17 (59%) had signs of ongoing renal injury. Of these 17, only 6 (35%) had ongoing nephrology follow-up.
- There were no differences in quality of life between study patients and healthy children.

STUDY CONCLUSIONS
There was a significant incidence of death and renal failure in children 3 to 5 years after AKI, and a high rate of residual renal injury even in ESRD-free survivors.

COMMENTARY
This study demonstrated for the first time that among children who survive hospitalizations with AKI, even with short-term normalization of renal function, there is a significant risk of subsequent mortality or renal failure. Ongoing renal injury was more prevalent than previously known, as demonstrated in the small subset of patients whom the authors reanalyzed. The study was limited by small sample size of patients within the reanalysis subgroup, but this does not diminish the powerful conclusions: AKI is a lasting morbidity rather than a short-term problem. Furthermore, this study emphasizes the importance of long-term follow-up with a pediatric nephrologist for children with AKI to assess and treat ongoing renal injury.

Question
AKI is known to be a prevalent and dangerous short-term complication in the inpatient setting, but what are the long-term outcomes?

Answer
In the months to years after hospitalization, these children are at high risk for progression of acute injury to chronic kidney disease, renal failure, and death.

Reference
1. Hui-Stickle S, Brewer ED, Goldstein SL. Pediatric ARF epidemiology at a tertiary care center from 1999 to 2001. *Am J Kidney Dis.* 2005;45(1):96–101.

CHAPTER 96

RESPONSE TO PREDNISONE IN NEPHROTIC SYNDROME

Michael Epstein ■ Avram Z. Traum

The Primary Nephrotic Syndrome in Children. Identification of Patients With Minimal Change Nephrotic Syndrome From Initial Response to Prednisone. A Report of the International Study of Kidney Disease in Children

J Pediatr. 1981;98(4):561–564

BACKGROUND
The prevalence of childhood nephrotic syndrome is 1:6,000.[1] Treatment and prognosis of primary nephrotic syndrome depend on cause, therefore early etiologic identification is a crucial step in management. Children with minimal change nephrotic syndrome (MCNS) can typically be managed with prednisone with an excellent prognosis, whereas children with other etiologies of nephrotic syndrome may require alternative therapies, progress to renal failure, or have other adverse outcomes. Common practice had been an initial corticosteroid trial with renal biopsy reserved only in those for whom this course failed. However, there was no supportive evidence and it was unclear if non-MCNS cases were being missed.

OBJECTIVES
To determine the predictive value of initial corticosteroid response in differentiating MCNS from other etiologies of primary nephrotic syndrome in children.

METHODS
Prospective cohort study at centers in the US, Canada, and Europe from 1967 to 1976.

Patients
471 children ages 12 weeks to 15 years meeting clinical criteria for nephrotic syndrome (proteinuria >40 mg/h/m^2, albumin <2.5 g/dL). Select exclusion criteria: prior exposure to corticosteroids, cytotoxic medications, or immunosuppressive agents.

Intervention
High-dose prednisone taper at an initial dose of 60 mg/m^2/d for 4 weeks, followed by 40 mg/m^2/d for 3 consecutive days per week for 4 weeks. All patients underwent renal biopsy prior to the initiation of therapy.

Outcomes
Primary outcome was reduction in proteinuria to 4 mg/h/m^2 (0 to trace on dipstick) for 3 consecutive days.

KEY RESULTS
- Nearly all patients with histopathologic MCNS (338/363, 93.1%) responded to initial corticosteroid therapy.
- Nearly all initial responders (338/368, 91.8%) were found on biopsy to have histopathologic MCNS.
- 87% of children ≤6 years old had MCNS, whereas only 53.2% of those >6 years had MCNS (p <0.05).
- When divided by age group, 47.9% of nonresponders ≤6 years had MCNS, whereas only 3.6% of nonresponders >6 years had MCNS.
- 93.8% of those who responded to corticosteroid treatment by 8 weeks had already responded at 4 weeks.

STUDY CONCLUSIONS
Corticosteroid response within 4 weeks, when positive, accurately predicted which children had MCNS, especially in children <6 years. However, corticosteroid nonresponse was less informative about diagnosis and prognosis, and should prompt renal biopsy.

COMMENTARY

This study validated the common practice of reserving renal biopsy in children with primary nephrotic syndrome until observing a response to an initial course of corticosteroids, under the assumption that nearly all responders will have MCNS and will have an excellent prognosis (a conclusion confirmed by long-term follow-up).[2] In doing so, it established an evidence-based standard of care still in practice today that reduces both potential harm and cost for most children with nephrotic syndrome. It also emphasized that nonresponders were likely to have other pathologies and should be referred for biopsy to guide care.

Question
Is response to an initial corticosteroid course predictive of etiology in children with primary nephrotic syndrome?

Answer
Initial corticosteroid response, when positive, accurately predicts which children have MCNS and can be spared a renal biopsy, especially in children <6 years old.

References
1. Eddy AA, Symons JM. Nephrotic syndrome in childhood. *Lancet.* 2003;362(9384):629–639.
2. Tarshish P, Tobin JN, Bernstein J, et al. Prognostic significance of the early course of minimal change nephrotic syndrome: Report of the International Study of Kidney Disease in Children. *J Am Soc Nephrol.* 1997;8(5):769–776.

RHEUMATOLOGY

97. Anakinra in Systemic Juvenile Idiopathic Arthritis
98. Treatment of Lupus With Mycophenolate Mofetil
99. Etanercept in Treatment of Juvenile Idiopathic Arthritis
100. Intravenous Immune Globulin for Kawasaki Disease

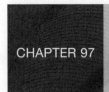

ANAKINRA IN SYSTEMIC JUVENILE IDIOPATHIC ARTHRITIS

Molly Miloslavsky ■ Eli Miloslavsky

A Multicentre, Randomised, Double-Blind, Placebo-Controlled Trial With the Interleukin-1 Receptor Antagonist Anakinra in Patients With Systemic-Onset Juvenile Idiopathic Arthritis (ANAJIS Trial)

Quartier P, Allantaz F, Cimaz R, et al. *Ann Rheum Dis.* 2011;70(5):747–754

BACKGROUND

Systemic juvenile idiopathic arthritis (SJIA) is characterized by arthritis, fevers, rash, and hepatosplenomegaly. Treatment options include nonsteroidal anti-inflammatory drugs (NSAIDs), corticosteroids, methotrexate, and anti-tumor necrosis factor agents, but some patients do not respond adequately. Insufficient treatment may lead to joint damage, macrophage activation syndrome, amyloidosis, and adverse effects from corticosteroids. There was evidence that interleukin-1 (IL-1) played an important role in the pathogenesis of SJIA; however, only several small case series demonstrated benefits of IL-1 blockade.

OBJECTIVES

To assess the efficacy of anakinra in treating patients with corticosteroid-dependent SJIA.

METHODS

Double-blind, randomized, placebo-controlled trial at 6 centers in France and the US.

Patients

24 patients ages 2 to 20 with SJIA for ≥6 months and active disease. Select exclusion criteria: prior anti–IL-1 treatment.

Intervention

Patients were randomized to receive anakinra 2 mg/kg/d (up to 100 mg) or placebo. Other immunosuppressive agents were discontinued. After 1 month, all patients could receive open-label anakinra and were followed for 12 months.

Outcomes

Primary outcome was the combination of American College of Rheumatology Pediatric (ACRpedi) 30 (a validated score measuring 30% improvement in at least 3/6 variables), resolution of fever, and 50% decreases in erythrocyte sedimentation rate (ESR) and C-reactive protein (CRP). Secondary outcomes were ACRpedi 50 and 70 (50% and 70% improvement) and safety and efficacy at 12 months.

KEY RESULTS

- At 1 month, 66% of patients in the anakinra group achieved ACRpedi 30 vs. 8% of patients in the control group ($p = 0.003$). 58% and 42% achieved ACRpedi 50 and 70, respectively, compared to none in the control group.
- Anakinra-treated patients had significantly lower ESR ($p = 0.002$) and CRP ($p = 0.001$) and fewer active joints ($p = 0.04$) compared to control group.
- Of the 16 patients who remained in the trial at 1 year, 43% remained responders, 38% were off prednisone, and 31% were in remission.
- There were no serious infections or differences in adverse events between groups.

STUDY CONCLUSIONS

Anakinra was effective in treating patients with SJIA, but there was a loss of response over time.

COMMENTARY

This study, in combination with several case series, led to the current recommendation that anakinra be used in patients with SJIA refractory to NSAIDs or corticosteroids and as first-line therapy in those with moderate or severe disease.[1] Use of anakinra and subsequent decreased corticosteroid use in this vulnerable patient population has been a major advancement. Study limitations included the small number of patients and relatively short duration of the double-blind phase. In cases of inadequate efficacy or loss of response to anakinra, recent trials have demonstrated that canakinumab (long acting anti–IL-1) and tocilizumab (anti–IL-6) can be effective.[2,3]

Question

Does anakinra have efficacy in treatment of SJIA?

Answer

Treatment with anakinra decreases disease activity and allows for corticosteroid tapering in SJIA.

References

1. Ringold S, Weiss PF, Beukelman T, et al. 2013 update of the 2011 American College of Rheumatology recommendations for the treatment of juvenile idiopathic arthritis: Recommendations for the medical therapy of children with systemic juvenile idiopathic arthritis and tuberculosis screening among children receiving biologic medications. *Arthritis Care and Res.* 2013;65(10):1551–1563.
2. Ruperto N, Brunner HI, Quartier P, et al. Two randomized trials of canakinumab in systemic juvenile idiopathic arthritis. *N Engl J Med.* 2012;367(25):2396–2406.
3. De Benedetti F, Brunner HI, Ruperto N, et al. Randomized trial of tocilizumab in systemic juvenile idiopathic arthritis. *N Engl J Med.* 2012;367(25):2385–2395.

CHAPTER 98

TREATMENT OF LUPUS WITH MYCOPHENOLATE MOFETIL

Molly Miloslavsky ■ Eli Miloslavsky

Mycophenolate Mofetil Treatment in Children and Adolescents With Lupus

Kazyra I, Pilkington C, Marks SD, Tullus K. *Arch Dis Child.* 2010;95(12):1059–1061

BACKGROUND

For severe manifestations of pediatric systemic lupus erythematosus (pSLE), including lupus nephritis, first line therapy has been the combination of corticosteroids with cyclophosphamide or azathioprine. However, prognosis remains poor and treatments have significant side effects. Studies in adults demonstrated that mycophenolate mofetil (MMF) was equivalent to cyclophosphamide in treating lupus nephritis; pediatric data were limited to small case series with heterogeneous disease manifestations.[1]

OBJECTIVES

To examine the safety and efficacy of MMF in pSLE.

METHODS

Retrospective study at 2 hospitals in the United Kingdom.

Patients

26 patients ages 5 to 18 years with pSLE; 23 were female and 18 had biopsy-proven lupus nephritis. Select exclusion criteria: none.

Intervention

MMF (target dose 20 to 25 mg/kg/d) in combination with corticosteroids (all patients) and hydroxychloroquine (16/26 patients). Patients in group 1 were started on MMF for induction or maintenance therapy (following induction with other medications). Group 2 was switched to MMF due to inadequate disease control with azathioprine. Patients were followed for 12 months.

Outcomes

Primary outcome was a change in the British Isles Lupus Assessment Group (BILAG) score (validated score based on signs and symptoms across 9 organ systems). Secondary outcomes included changes in renal function, auto-antibodies, and hematologic parameters.

KEY RESULTS

- The BILAG score improved in 77% (20/26) of patients across both groups (9 to 3, $p < 0.05$).
- In patients with lupus nephritis, including the 2 patients who received MMF as induction therapy, there was significant improvement in renal function and proteinuria.

- MMF permitted corticosteroid tapering in both groups (25 to 6.5 mg in group 1 and 15 to 5 mg in group 2, p <0.05).
- In group 1, significant improvements were seen in hemoglobin (9.7 to 12.6 g/dL, p <0.05), ESR (63 to 16 mm/h, p <0.05), and lymphocyte count (0.57 × 10^9/L to 1.71 × 10^9/L, p <0.05).
- 4 patients experienced adverse effects, none of which resulted in discontinuation of therapy.

STUDY CONCLUSIONS

MMF appeared to be a safe and effective treatment for pSLE.

COMMENTARY

This was the largest study to date demonstrating the safety and efficacy of MMF in pSLE. Despite significant limitations such as the retrospective design, heterogeneous patient population, and prior treatment with various agents, it helped pave the way for the use of MMF in pSLE, particularly in patients with nephritis.[2] This was supported by the need for agents with less potential toxicity than cyclophosphamide and adult data from lupus nephritis trials demonstrating MMF's equivalence. However, some pediatric providers continue to use cyclophosphamide due to MMF's limited evidence base in children. Further studies are needed in children with lupus nephritis as well as those with neurologic and hematologic involvement.

Question

Is treatment with MMF beneficial in children and adolescents with lupus?

Answer

Yes, MMF appears to have efficacy in pSLE, particularly in patients with nephritis.

References

1. Appel GB, Contreras G, Dooley MA, et al. Mycophenolate mofetil versus cyclophosphamide for induction treatment of lupus nephritis. *J Am Soc Nephrol.* 2009;20(5):1103–1112.
2. Tullus K. New developments in the treatment of systemic lupus erythematosus. *Pediatr Nephrol.* 2012; 27(5):727–732.

CHAPTER 99

ETANERCEPT IN TREATMENT OF JUVENILE IDIOPATHIC ARTHRITIS

Molly Miloslavsky ■ Eli Miloslavsky

Etanercept in Children With Polyarticular Juvenile Rheumatoid Arthritis. Pediatric Rheumatology Collaborative Study Group

Lovell DJ, Giannini EH, Reiff A, et al. *N Engl J Med.* 2000;342(11):763–769

BACKGROUND

Juvenile idiopathic arthritis (JIA) is the most common type of arthritis in children and can lead to significant functional impairment. Methotrexate had been the mainstay of treatment when nonsteroidal anti-inflammatory drugs (NSAIDs) were insufficient; however, a significant percentage of patients did not achieve disease control with these agents. Tumor necrosis factor (TNF) is a proinflammatory cytokine implicated in the pathogenesis of JIA. Anti-TNF agents, such as etanercept, had been shown to be effective for rheumatoid arthritis in the adult population, but pediatric data were lacking.

OBJECTIVES

To evaluate the safety and efficacy of etanercept in children with polyarticular JIA refractory to methotrexate.

METHODS

Double-blind, randomized, placebo-controlled trial at 10 centers in the US and Canada.

Patients

69 patients ages 4 to 17 years with active polyarticular arthritis (≥5 joints) with inadequate response to methotrexate. Select exclusion criteria: pregnancy, lactation.

Intervention

Open-label phase: all patients received etanercept (0.4 mg/kg, up to 25 mg) twice weekly for up to 3 months. Randomized double-blind phase: patients who improved either continued to receive etanercept or received placebo for 4 months, unless disease flare occurred. Methotrexate was discontinued but stable doses of NSAIDs or corticosteroids were allowed. Disease activity was evaluated every 2 weeks.

Outcomes

Open-label phase: percentage of patients achieving American College of Rheumatology pediatric (ACRpedi) 30, 50, and 70 (a validated score measuring improvement by 30%, 50%, and 70% in multiple variables). Double-blind phase: number of patients with disease flare.

KEY RESULTS

- 74% (51/69) of patients reached ACRpedi 30 on etanercept in the open-label phase.
- Once randomized, etanercept-treated patients had significantly fewer flares compared to those in the placebo group: 28% (7/25) vs. 81% (21/26), $p = 0.003$.
- At 7 months, 80% (20/25) of patients receiving etanercept achieved ACRpedi 30, 72% (18/25) achieved ACRpedi 50, and 44% (11/25) achieved ACRpedi 70 vs. 35% (9/26), 23% (6/26), and 19% (5/26), respectively in the placebo group.
- There were no differences in adverse events between groups.

STUDY CONCLUSIONS

Etanercept was well tolerated and significantly decreased disease activity in pediatric patients with polyarticular JIA compared to placebo.

COMMENTARY

This industry-sponsored study was the first to demonstrate the benefit of TNF inhibition in children with methotrexate-refractory polyarticular JIA. Subsequent studies also demonstrated similar benefit in patients with oligoarticular JIA, prompting consensus guidelines to recommend TNF inhibitors in patients with incomplete disease control with NSAIDs and methotrexate.[1] Notably, patients with systemic JIA were included in this study, however studies have shown that such patients respond better to interleukin-1 and interleukin-6 inhibition.[2] Approximately 20% to 25% of patients with JIA do not obtain sufficient benefit from etanercept; such patients may benefit from switching to another TNF inhibitor.[3]

Question

Is etanercept a safe and effective agent in polyarticular JIA?

Answer

Yes. Etanercept leads to significant improvement in JIA refractory to methotrexate.

References

1. Beukelman T, Patkar NM, Saag KG, et al. 2011 American College of Rheumatology recommendations for the treatment of juvenile idiopathic arthritis: Initiation and safety monitoring of therapeutic agents for the treatment of arthritis and systemic features. *Arthritis Care Res (Hoboken).* 2011;63(4):465–482.
2. Ringold S, Weiss PF, Beukelman T, et al. 2013 update of the 2011 American College of Rheumatology recommendations for the treatment of juvenile idiopathic arthritis: Recommendations for the medical therapy of children with systemic juvenile idiopathic arthritis and tuberculosis screening among children receiving biologic medications. *Arthritis Care Res (Hoboken).* 2013;65(10):1551–1563.
3. Otten MH, Prince FH, Anink J, et al. Effectiveness and safety of a second and third biological agent after failing etanercept in juvenile idiopathic arthritis: Results from the Dutch National ABC Register. *Ann Rheum Dis.* 2013;72(5):721–727.

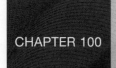

INTRAVENOUS IMMUNE GLOBULIN FOR KAWASAKI DISEASE

CHAPTER 100

Molly Miloslavsky ■ Eli Miloslavsky

The Treatment of Kawasaki Syndrome With Intravenous Gamma Globulin
Newburger JW, Takahashi M, Burns JC, et al. *N Engl J Med.* 1986;315(6):341–347

BACKGROUND

Kawasaki disease (KD) is a medium-vessel vasculitis that primarily affects children under the age of 5, and is one of the leading causes of acquired pediatric heart disease. Due to its anti-inflammatory effects, aspirin had been the mainstay of therapy although it had not been shown to prevent the development of coronary artery aneurysms. An unblinded study from Japan demonstrated that IV immune globulin (IVIG) may prevent development of coronary artery lesions in children with KD but no randomized trials had been conducted.[1]

OBJECTIVES

To compare aspirin alone vs. aspirin plus IVIG in preventing coronary artery aneurysms in children with KD.

METHODS

Randomized controlled trial in 6 US hospitals from 1984 to 1985.

Patients

168 children (mean age 2.5 years) who met at least 5/6 inclusion criteria: fever, nonexudative conjunctivitis, oropharyngeal changes (strawberry tongue, dry fissured lips, and mucosal erythema), changes in extremities (erythema of palms/soles, edema of hands/feet), rash, and cervical lymphadenopathy. Select exclusion criteria: symptoms >10 days.

Intervention

Patients were randomized to aspirin alone (100 mg/kg/d for 2 weeks, then 3 to 5 mg/kg/d) or similarly dosed aspirin plus IVIG (400 mg/kg/d for 4 days).

Outcomes

Primary outcomes were presence of coronary artery abnormalities at 2 and 7 weeks after enrollment as diagnosed by blinded echocardiograms. Secondary outcomes included duration of fever and changes in inflammatory markers.

KEY RESULTS

- Patients treated with IVIG had fewer coronary artery abnormalities than those treated with aspirin alone: 8% vs. 23% ($p = 0.01$) and 4% vs. 18% ($p = 0.005$), at 2 and 7 weeks, respectively.

- Patients in the IVIG group were more likely to be afebrile on day 2 of the study (86% vs. 46%, p <0.01) and had more rapid improvements in white blood cell count ($p = 0.0001$) and absolute granulocyte count ($p = 0.0001$).
- Adverse events included mild congestive heart failure (3 patients in the IVIG group and 4 patients in the aspirin group) and sepsis (1 patient in the IVIG group).

STUDY CONCLUSIONS

IVIG administered in conjunction with aspirin early in the disease course was well-tolerated and produced greater improvement in laboratory abnormalities, faster defervescence, and decreased coronary artery abnormalities in children with KD.

COMMENTARY

This study led to IVIG, in combination with aspirin, becoming the standard of care for KD. More recent studies have demonstrated that a single higher dose of IVIG (2 g/kg) is more effective than the dosing used in this study.[2] It is recommended that treatment be started within the first 7 days of illness in order to prevent the development of coronary lesions; however, this remains a challenging clinical diagnosis. For patients who remain febrile after the first dose, most experts recommend repeat IVIG.[3] Other agents such as corticosteroids and infliximab are under investigation as potential therapies in patients with refractory KD.

Question

Does IVIG reduce the incidence of coronary artery abnormalities in children with KD?

Answer

Yes. IVIG reduces the risk of developing coronary artery aneurysms if administered early in the disease course.

References

1. Furusho K, Kamiya T, Nakano H, et al. High-dose intravenous gammaglobulin for Kawasaki disease. *Lancet.* 1984;2(8411):1055–1058.
2. Terai M, Shulman ST. Prevalence of coronary artery abnormalities in Kawasaki disease is highly dependent on gamma globulin dose but independent of salicylate dose. *J Pediatr.* 1997;131(6):888–893.
3. Newburger JW, Takahashi M, Gerber MA, et al. Diagnosis, treatment, and long-term management of Kawasaki disease: A statement for health professionals from the Committee on Rheumatic Fever, Endocarditis, and Kawasaki Disease, Council on Cardiovascular Disease in the Young, American Heart Association. *Pediatrics.* 2004;114(6):1708–1733.

INDEX

Note: Page number followed by f and t indicate figure and table only.

A

AAP. *See* American Academy of Pediatrics
Absolute neutrophil count (ANC), and risk of appendicitis, 46–47
Acute kidney injury (AKI), 226
  mortality associated with, 226–227
  outcomes after, 230–231
  RIFLE criteria, 226–227
Acute lung injury (ALI), low tidal volume ventilation in, 40–41
Acute lymphoblastic leukemia (ALL), minimal residual disease and, 110–111
Acute otitis media (AOM)
  amoxicillin-clavulanate for, 176–177
  severity of symptoms scale, 176, 177
  treatment of, 176–177
Acute respiratory distress syndrome (ARDS)
  low tidal volume (TV) ventilation in, 40–41
  traditional TV ventilation in, 40–41
Acyclovir, high doses, for neonatal HSV disease, 132–133
Adenotonsillectomy, for obstructive sleep apnea, 206–207
Adolescents
  contraceptive counseling for, 174
  long-acting reversible contraceptive by, use of, 174–175
  major depressive disorder in, combination therapy for, 192–193
  sexually transmitted infections in, prevalence of, 180–181
  teenage pregnancy rate, reduction in, 174–175
Adult survivors, of pediatric cancer, 112–113
Adverse childhood experiences (ACEs), role of, on long-term health outcomes, 198–199
AEDs. *See* Antiepileptic drugs
AKI. *See* Acute kidney injury
Albuterol
  for asthma, 62–63
  for bronchiolitis, 214–215
Allergy
  cow's milk, 6–7
  egg, 2–3
  peanut, 8–9
American Academy of Pediatrics (AAP), 52, 56, 119, 133, 137, 139, 159, 176, 181, 189, 215
Amitriptyline, for pediatric headaches, 168–169
Amoxicillin-clavulanate, for acute otitis media, 176–177

Anakinra, in systemic-onset juvenile idiopathic arthritis, 236–237
Angiotensin II receptor blockers (ARBs), in Marfan syndrome, 100–101
Antibiotics
  for acute otitis media, 176–177
  after incision and drainage of skin abscesses, 124–125
  for osteomyelitis, 126–127
  pretreatment on cerebrospinal fluid profiles, effect of, 128–129
  for sepsis, 28–29
  for urinary tract infections, 136–137
  for vesicoureteral reflux, 224–225
Antiepileptic drugs (AEDs)
  cessation of, predictors of, 163
  seizure recurrence after withdrawal of, 162–163
Antiretroviral drugs, for preventing mother-to-child transmission of HIV, 140–141
AOM. *See* Acute otitis media
AOP. *See* Apnea of prematurity
Aortic dilation in Marfan syndrome, effect of ARBs on, 100–101
Aortic valvuloplasty, and hypoplastic left heart syndrome, 20–21
Apnea of prematurity (AOP), 146
  caffeine for, 146–147
Appendicitis, prediction rule for, 46–47
ARDS. *See* Acute respiratory distress syndrome
Asthma
  budesonide in, 210–211
  inhaled corticosteroids in, 210–211
  ipratropium in, 62–63
  oral corticosteroids in, 212–213
  wheezing and risk of, 220–221
Attention deficit hyperactivity disorder (ADHD), combination treatment for, 194–196
Autism spectrum disorder (ASD)
  behavioral therapy for, 202–203
  and MMR vaccine, association between, 186–187

B

BABY HUG trial, 117
Back-to-Sleep campaign, 189
Bacterial infections, in RSV-positive infants, 130–131

Bacterial meningitis
antibiotic pretreatment effect on CSF profiles in, 128–129
and first simple febrile seizure, 52–53
Behavioral therapy
for attention deficit hyperactivity disorder, 194–196
for autism, 202–203
Beta-agonist therapy, route of delivery of, 218–219
Bhutani nomogram, 155f, 156
Bicarbonate therapy, and cerebral edema in DKA, 75
Bilirubin screening, in neonates, 154–156, 155f
Biphasic anaphylactic reactions, in children, 10–11
epinephrine administration and, 11
Blood pressure control, impact of, on progression of renal failure, 228–229
Blood transfusions
restrictive protocol for, 38–39
for stroke prevention in sickle cell anemia, 120–121
Body mass index (BMI), elevated, and pubertal development, 72–73
British Isles Lupus Assessment Group (BILAG) score, 238
Bronchiolitis
high-flow nasal cannula therapy for, 34–35
management of, 214–215
Bronchopulmonary dysplasia (BPD), caffeine therapy and, 146–147
Budesonide, in persistent mild asthma, 210–211
Bystander cardiopulmonary resuscitation (CPR), in pediatric out-of-hospital cardiac arrests, 36–37

C
Caffeine therapy, for apnea of prematurity, 146–147
Canakinumab, 237
Cancer survivors, chronic disease in, 112–113
Cardiopulmonary resuscitation (CPR), 36–37
Cardiovascular disease (CVD), childhood obesity and, 178–179
Celiac disease (CD), 82
genetic susceptibility to, 82
prevalence of, 88–89
timing of gluten introduction on, impact of, 82–83
Cell-free DNA (cfDNA) technology, for T21 screening, 96–97
Centers for Disease Control and Prevention (CDC), 151, 175, 184

Central venous catheters (CVCs), 32–33
Cerebral edema, diabetic ketoacidosis and, 74–75
Cerebrospinal fluid (CSF) sampling, effect of antibiotic pretreatment on, 128–129
CF. *See* Cystic fibrosis
CH. *See* Congenital hypothyroidism
CHD. *See* Congenital heart disease
Chest pain (CP)
algorithm for evaluation, 16f
and cardiac disease in children, 15
causes of, 14–15
Chest radiographs (CXRs), in febrile children with leukocytosis, 60–61
Childhood abuse and household dysfunction, and health outcomes in adulthood, 198–199
Childhood and Adolescent Migraine Prevention (CHAMP) study, 169
Childhood Cancer Survivor Study (CCSS), 112–113
Childhood obesity and cardiovascular risk, 178–179
Children's Depression Rating Scale-Revised (CDRS-R) score, 192
Chlamydia screening, for sexually active females, 181
Clinical Global Assessment (CGI) score, 192, 193
Cognitive-behavioral therapy (CBT), for adolescent depression, 192–193
Community-acquired MRSA (CA-MRSA), treatment of, 124–125
Community-acquired skin abscesses, management of, 124–125
Compression-only cardiopulmonary resuscitation (COCPR), 36–37
Congenital heart disease (CHD)
pulse oximetry screening for, 18–19
repair of, in low birth weight (LBW) infants, 22–23
Congenital hypothyroidism (CH)
and intellectual impairment, 78–79
newborn screening for, 78–79
untreated, 78
Conners Rating Scale, 207
Constipation, polyethylene glycol for, 90–91
Continuous positive airway pressure (CPAP), 34, 159
Corticosteroids
for asthma, 62–63
for croup, 58–59
for idiopathic thrombocytopenic purpura, 114–115
inhaled, in persistent mild asthma, 210–211
for nephrotic syndrome, 232–233
oral, in asthma exacerbations, 212–213

Cough, upper respiratory tract infections and, 182–183
Cow's milk allergy (CMA), IgE-mediated, resolution of, 6–7
CPR. *See* Cardiopulmonary resuscitation
Crohn disease, infliximab therapy for, 86–87
CT scan, in head trauma, 48–49
Cystic fibrosis (CF), 216
  early diagnosis of, 216–217
  hypertonic saline in, 208–209
  neonatal screening for, 216–217

D
Depression, combination therapy for, 192–193
Developmental outcomes
  low-level lead exposure and, 184–185
  preterm birth and, 164–165
Dexamethasone, in mild croup, 58–59
Dextromethorphan (DM), for nocturnal cough, 182–183
Diabetes Control and Complications Trial (DCCT), 77
Diabetic ketoacidosis (DKA), and cerebral edema, 74–75
Diphenhydramine (DPH), for nocturnal cough, 182–183

E
Early intervention (EI) programs, for preterm infants, 200–201
Egg allergy, oral immunotherapy for, 2–3
End of life care, in pediatric oncology, 118–119
The Epidemiology of Diabetes Interventions and Complications (EDIC) study, 77
Epilepsy, seizure recurrence after AED withdrawal in, 162–163
Epinephrine, for bronchiolitis, 214–215
Etanercept, in juvenile idiopathic arthritis, 240–241
European Society of Hypertension, 229

F
Factor VIII (FVIII) infusions, in hemophilia, 108–109
Febrile infants, evaluation and management of, 64–67
  Boston study, 64t–66t, 66
  Philadelphia study, 64t–66t, 66–67
  Rochester study, 64t–66t, 66
Febrile seizure, risk of unprovoked seizures after, 170–171
Fetal aortic valve stenosis with evolving hypoplastic left heart syndrome, prenatal echocardiograms for, 20–21
First simple febrile seizure (FSFS), lumbar puncture in, 52–53

Fluid resuscitation, in pediatric septic shock, 42–43

G
Gastroenteritis
  oral ondansetron for, 54–55
  oral rehydration *vs.* intravenous rehydration, 56–57
GBS disease. *See* Group B streptococcal (GBS) disease
Genetic disorders, whole-exome sequencing for, 94–95
Glycemic control, in type 2 diabetes, 70–71
Group B streptococcal (GBS) disease
  early-onset, prevention of, 150–151
  universal screening for, during pregnancy, 150–151

H
Headache, 168
  amitriptyline for, 168–169
  isolated chronic, serious intracranial pathology in, 166–167
Head trauma
  and clinically important traumatic brain injury (ciTBI), 48–49, 50f
  CT scan in, 48–49
Healthy Steps program, 199
Hemophilia A, prophylactic factor VIII (FVIII) infusions in, 108–109
Herpes simplex virus (HSV) infection, high-dose acyclovir for, 132–133
HIE. *See* Hypoxic-ischemic encephalopathy
High-flow nasal cannula (HFNC) therapy, in bronchiolitis, 34–35
Honey, for cough, 183
Human immunodeficiency virus (HIV), perinatal transmission of, reduction of, 140–141
Human papillomavirus (HPV) vaccination, in preadolescence, 181
Hydroxyurea, in sickle cell anemia, 116–117
Hyperbilirubinemia, in infants, 154–156, 155f
Hypertonic saline (HTS), in cystic fibrosis, 208–209
Hypoplastic left heart syndrome (HLHS), fetal aortic valve stenosis and, 20–21
Hypoxic-ischemic encephalopathy (HIE)
  neonatal brain injury, 148
  therapeutic hypothermia in, 148–149

I
Idiopathic thrombocytopenic purpura (ITP)
  American Society of Hematology recommendations, 115
  treatment of, 114–115

Inborn errors of metabolism (IEM), mass
  spectrometry screening for, 98–99
Incision and drainage (I&D), of skin abscesses,
  124–125
Individuals with Disabilities Education Act,
  1987, 200
Infliximab
  in pediatric Crohn disease, 86–87
  in steroid-refractory ulcerative colitis, 85
Inhaled corticosteroids, in persistent mild
  asthma, 210–211
Insulin therapy, intensive, for type 1 diabetes
  mellitus, 76–77
Intellectual impairment
  congenital hypothyroidism and, 78–79
  low-level lead exposure and, 184–185
Intelligence quotient (IQ)
  low-level lead exposure and, 184–185
  preterm infants and, 164–165
Intrauterine devices (IUDs), 174
Intravenous rehydration *vs.* oral rehydration,
  56–57
Intraventricular hemorrhages (IVHs),
  prematurity-associated, and
  neurodevelopmental outcomes, 164–165
In utero aortic valvuloplasty, and hypoplastic left
  heart syndrome, 20–21
Ipratropium, in pediatric asthma, 62–63
IQ. *See* Intelligence quotient
Isolated chronic headache, in children, 166–167
ITP. *See* Idiopathic thrombocytopenic purpura
IV immune globulin (IVIG)
  for idiopathic thrombocytopenic purpura,
  114–115
  for Kawasaki disease, 242–243

J
Joint disease in hemophilia, prevention of,
  108–109
Juvenile idiopathic arthritis (JIA), etanercept in,
  240–241

K
Kawasaki disease (KD), IV immunoglobulin for,
  242–243

L
Laryngotracheobronchitis, oral dexamethasone
  for, 58–59
Lead exposure, low-level, effect on intellectual
  impairment, 184–185
Levothyroxine, for subclinical congenital
  hypothyroidism, 79
Long-acting reversible contraception (LARC),
  use of, by adolescents, 174–175

Low-birth-weight (LBW) infants
  CHD repair in, 22–23
  early developmental intervention for, 200–201
Lower tidal volume (TV) ventilation, in acute
  respiratory distress syndrome, 40–41
Lumbar puncture (LP), in children with first
  simple febrile seizure, 52–53

M
Major depressive disorder (MDD) in
  adolescents, combination therapy for,
  192–193
Marfan syndrome, angiotensin receptor blockers
  in, 100–101
Massively parallel sequencing (MPS) technology,
  96
  for T21 screening, 96–97
Measles, mumps, and rubella (MMR) vaccine
  and autism, association between, 186–187
Meconium-stained neonates, management of,
  152–153
Medulloblastoma, genetic predictors of outcome
  in, 104–106, 105f
Metered-dose inhalers (MDIs) with spacers, for
  wheezing, 218–219
Metformin, for type 2 diabetes mellitus, 70–71
Methicillin-resistant Staphylococcus aureus
  (MRSA) infection, in children, 124–125
Methylxanthines, for apnea of prematurity, 146
Migraine, amitriptyline for, 168–169
Minimal change nephrotic syndrome (MCNS),
  prednisone in, 232–233
Minimal residual disease (MRD), and acute
  lymphoblastic leukemia, 110–111
Molecular markers, in medulloblastoma, 104–
  106, 105f
Mother-to-child transmission (MTCT), of
  human immunodeficiency virus, 140–141
Mycophenolate mofetil (MMF), for pediatric
  systemic lupus erythematosus (pSLE),
  238–239

N
National Asthma Education and Prevention
  Program, 211
Neonatal herpes simplex virus (HSV) infection,
  IV acyclovir (ACV) for, 132–133
Neonatal jaundice, postdischarge, 154–156, 155f
Neonatal screening, for hypothyroidism, 78–79
Nephrotic syndrome, prednisone response in,
  232–233
Neuroimaging, in children with headache,
  166–167
Nevirapine, for prevention of MTCT, 141
Normal saline, for bronchiolitis, 214–215

O
Obesity in childhood, 178
and CVD risk factors in adulthood, 178–179
Obstructive sleep apnea (OSA), 206
adenotonsillectomy for, 206–207
risk factor for, 206
Occult pneumonia, in febrile children, 60–61
Ondansetron, for gastroenteritis, 54–55
Oral immunotherapy (OIT), for egg allergy, 2–3
Oral rehydration therapy (ORT), 54–55
vs. intravenous rehydration, 56–57
ORT. See Oral rehydration therapy
OSA. See Obstructive sleep apnea
Osteomyelitis, sequential therapy for, 126–127
Over-the-counter (OTC) cold medications, for
nocturnal cough, 182–183

P
Palivizumab, for respiratory syncytial virus
infections, 138–139
Palliative care programs, for children with
cancer, 119
Peanut allergy, natural history of, 8–9
Pediatric intensive care unit (PICU)
antimicrobial therapy in sepsis in, 28–29
CVC care bundles use in, 32–33
daily sedation breaks in, 30–31
transfusion strategies for patients in, 38–39
Pediatric oncology, end of life needs in, study on,
118–119
Pediatric sepsis, early antibiotic administration
in, 28–29
Pediatric Ulcerative Colitis Activity Index
(PUCAI), 84–85
PICU. See Pediatric intensive care unit
PID. See Primary immunodeficiency diseases
Polyethylene glycol 3350 (PEG), for
constipation, 90–91
Polysomnographic (PSG) testing, 206–207
Preterm birth, effect of, on long-term
developmental outcomes, 164–165
Preterm infants
early intervention (EI) programs for, 200–201
extremely, predictors for survival in, 144–145
Primary immunodeficiency diseases (PID)
B-cell, 5
clinical identification of, 4–5
failure to thrive and, 5
family history of, 5
IV antibiotics needs to treat infections in, 5
warning signs of, 4
Prone sleeping position, and risk of SUID,
188–189
Pubertal development, body mass index and,
72–73

PUCAI. See Pediatric Ulcerative Colitis Activity
Index
Pulse oximetry screening, for congenital heart
defects in newborns, 18–19

R
Reflux nephropathy, 224
Renal failure in children, impact of blood
pressure control on, 228–229
Respiratory distress syndrome (RDS), surfactant
therapy in, 158–159
Respiratory syncytial virus (RSV), 130
palivizumab for prophylaxis against, 138–139
Restrictive transfusion strategy, in pediatrics,
38–39
Resuscitation, of extremely premature infant, 145
Rosiglitazone, for type 2 diabetes mellitus,
70–71
RSV. See Respiratory syncytial virus
RSV IV immunoglobulin (RSV-IVIG), 138
RSV-positive infants, serious bacterial infections
(SBIs) in, 130–131

S
SCA. See Sickle cell anemia
Sedation interruption, in intubated children,
30–31
Seizure recurrence risk, after AED withdrawal,
162–163
Selective serotonin reuptake inhibitors (SSRIs),
for adolescent depression, 192–193
Sepsis, early antibiotic administration in, 28–29
Septic arthritis (SA) and transient synovitis,
distinction between, 134–135
Septic shock, early fluid resuscitation in, 42–43
Sequential therapy, for osteomyelitis, 126–127
Serious bacterial infection (SBI), in infants, 64–65
Sexually transmitted infections (STIs),
prevalence of, in adolescent females,
180–181
Sickle cell anemia (SCA)
hydroxyurea in, 116–117
stroke risk reduction in, 120–121
SJIA. See Systemic-onset juvenile idiopathic
arthritis
Stacked nebulizer treatments, for acute asthma,
63
STOP2 trial, 121
Stroke prevention, in sickle cell anemia, 120–121
Sudden death, in young athletes, 24–25
cardiovascular cause of, 24–25
preparticipation cardiovascular screening for
prevention of, 26t
Sudden infant death syndrome (SIDS). See
Sudden unexpected infant death

Sudden unexpected infant death (SUID), sleep position and, 188–189
Surfactant, in respiratory distress syndrome, 158–159
Surviving Sepsis Campaign, 28
Systemic lupus erythematosus, mycophenolate mofetil in, 238–239
Systemic-onset juvenile idiopathic arthritis (SJIA), 236
anakinra in, 236–237
treatment of, 236

T
Tandem mass spectrometry (TMS), for inborn errors of metabolism, 98–99
T1DM. *See* Type 1 diabetes mellitus
T2DM. *See* Type 2 diabetes mellitus
Therapeutic hypothermia, for infants with HIE, 148–149
Tocilizumab, 237
Total serum bilirubin (TSB) screening, predischarge, 154–156, 155f
Transcranial Doppler ultrasonography (TCD), for stroke prevention in sickle cell anemia, 120–121
Transfusion strategy, restrictive *vs* liberal, in pediatrics, 38–39
Transient synovitis (TS) and septic arthritis, distinction between, 134–135
Treatment for Adolescents With Depression Study (TADS), 192–193
Trisomy 21 (T21), 96
noninvasive prenatal testing for, 96–97
Type 1 diabetes mellitus (T1DM)
complications of, 76
intensive insulin treatment for, 76–77
Type 2 diabetes mellitus (T2DM), 70
glycemic control in, 70–71
TODAY study, 71

U
UC. *See* Ulcerative colitis
Ulcerative colitis (UC), 84
PUCAI score in, use of, 84–85
salvage therapy for, 84–85
steroid-refractory, 84
Urinary tract infections (UTIs)
oral *vs* intravenous therapy for, 136–137
in RSV-positive infants, 130–131
vesicoureteral reflux and, 224–225
UTIs. *See* Urinary tract infections

V
Very low–birth-weight (VLBW) newborns, caffeine therapy in, 146–147
Vesicoureteral reflux (VUR)
antibiotic prophylaxis in, 224–225
and urinary tract infections, 224
Viral bronchiolitis, 214–215
Vomiting, during oral rehydration therapy, 54–55
VUR. *See* Vesicoureteral reflux

W
Weight, impact of, on outcomes of CHD repair, 22–23
WES. *See* Whole-exome sequencing
Wheezing
nebulizers *vs.* metered-dose inhalers in, 218–219
risk of asthma, 220–221
Whole-body hypothermia, for neonatal HIE, 148–149
Whole-exome sequencing (WES), 94–95
World Health Organization (WHO), 56, 184

Z
Zidovudine (AZT), for reduction of perinatal transmission of HIV, 140–141